# Losing My Kidney and Finding My Voice

## Confessions of a Living Donor

By Rachel Bennett Steury

*To the world you may be one person,
but to one person, you may be the world."
— Dr. Seuss*

# Reader Reviews

"This book offers a fascinating and enjoyable look into a world that most people do not even know exists. It shows you this world from the point of view of an ordinary person discovering it for the first time."

Dan Cragan
Playwright, composer, kidney and pancreas transplant recipient

"Rachel is the real deal. A genuine generous heart, she does the research to meet her goals, one of which was to start a chain by donating her kidney. A later goal was to write a book about it. For such a private person, Rachel opens up about her family history, her current family, friends, and colleagues, and her place in the world — and the actions she's willing to take to change the world. I want to be like Rachel — you will too!"

Beth Berry
Author of *Haiku Frenzy*, endometrial and kidney cancer survivor

"Well now, here's a present-day antidote for — as Thomas Paine once put it — "the times that try men's souls". Rachel writes about her quintessentially human journey toward a brighter tomorrow. Her memoir is well-written and memorable on its own as a story of self-discovery, but its depth is profoundly spiritual. An inspiration during our troubled times."

Denning Powell
Co-Author of the Science Fiction Trilogy
*Monkey Trap*, *Hiding Hand*, and *Splintered Light*

**Losing My Kidney and Finding My Voice**
Confessions of a Living Donor

Author: Rachel Bennett Steury
Editor: Brenda E. Cortez
Interior Layout: Michael Nicloy
Cover Design: Brad Cawley-Hamm
Cover Photo Credits:
  Meghan Hasse, Silhouette Image
  Mathew Steury, Technical Support
  Georgia Cawley, Creative Consultant

Published by: BC Books, LLC
Franklin, Wisconsin
Brenda E. Cortez, Publisher
bcbooksllc.com
Info@bcbooksllc.com

Printed in The United States of America

**Names:** Steury, Rachel Bennett, author. | Brooks, Edwin (Ned), writer of foreword. | Johnson, J. Randy, writer of afterword.
**Title:** Losing my kidney and finding my voice : confessions of a living donor / by Rachel Bennett Steury.
**Description:** Franklin, Wisconsin : BC Books, LLC, [2026] | Includes bibliographical references.
**Identifiers:** ISBN: 9798990720589 (Paperback) | 9798995008705 (Ebook) | 9798234011688 (Audiobook)
**Subjects:** LCSH: Organ donors--Psychology. | Donation of organs, tissues, etc.--Psychological aspects. | Transplantation of organs, tissues, etc. | Kidneys--Transplantation. | Kidneys--Transplantation--Patients--United States. | LCGFT: Autobiographies.
**Classification:** LCC: RD129.5 .S74 2026 | DDC: 617.4/610592--dc23

Paperback ISBN: 979-8-9907205-8-9
Paperback: Human Authored™, Reg #: 1196187, _authorsguild.org/human_

Ebook ISBN: 979-8-9950087-0-5
Ebook: Human Authored™, Reg #: 1703129, _authorsguild.org/human_

AudioBook ISBN: ISBN 979-8-234-01168-8
Human Authored™ Reg #: 8113141, _authorsguild.org/human_

# **Dedication**

This book is dedicated to the matriarch of our family, Barbara Jean Laux, also known as Grana. Grana lived a long life of rolling with the punches. I'll forever remember her resilience and be grateful for her unconditional love.

# Table of Contents

# Foreword

## by Ned Brooks

## Founder, National Kidney Donation Organization

Each year, roughly one in a million Americans, approximately 300 to 450, donate a kidney to a stranger. The term for such a donation has several names — "altruistic donor," "non-directed donor" (often shortened to "NDD"), "good Samaritan donor" are a few of them. The problem with the term "altruistic donor" is that someone who donates a kidney to a loved one or an acquaintance can, justifiably, take issue with the insinuation that their donation is not altruistic. I prefer the term non-directed donor, or NDD, since it simply states a fact.

The conundrum which Rachel explores in this book is one with which I, along with almost every other NDD of my acquaintance, have wrestled at some length. For us, the decision to donate a kidney was mostly straightforward. The asymmetry of the transaction is stark: a few days of discomfort for the donor in return for dramatically altering the life trajectory of both a person with renal failure and their entire family. Every NDD I have met, at some point in our conversation, admits that they do not view themselves as a hero or someone who has made a great sacrifice. We are genuinely baffled by the heroic descriptions others insist on labeling us with. But the numbers tell us we are special, we are one in a million. Why? How is it possible that over 700,000 Americans can languish on dialysis, with over 90,000 on the waitlist approved for a transplant, and only one in a million people come forward to do something that we, the ones who speak from experience, largely consider a minor inconvenience?

Obviously, or at least obvious to me, NDDs are wired differently. Abigail Marsh is a Professor of Psychology at Georgetown University and the world's leading expert on the study of the psychology and physiology of non-directed donors. It is her contention that NDDs have an enlarged amygdala, a pair of organs in the brain that are involved in emotional regulation, memory, and behavioral responses. Someone with a larger amygdala tends to empathize more deeply with people who are outside the circle of family and friends, for whom the average person may be more inclined to make a sacrifice. If Professor Marsh is correct, that may account for what we NDDs call "the lightning strike"; that moment of clarity when we knew in an instant that this is something we both want to do and, for many of us, we feel compelled to do.

A word on altruism. This is part and parcel of the conundrum — is someone who donates a kidney to a stranger really an altruist? Philosophers and theologians have explored the nature of altruism to a fare-thee-well. I remain suspect. Stephen Dubner, an economist and co-author of the Freakonomics books and podcast empire, speaks about the "warm glow" that accrues to someone who acts in a way we commonly term "altruistic." That warm glow may be considered sufficient compensation, which obviates the "altruist" label. I know this is quite true in my case; I spend a fair amount of time counseling both donor candidates and patients seeking a kidney donor. Someone asked me just the other day why I do this, and I gave him the simple answer—it's a lot of fun for me and gives me great satisfaction. I am well compensated.

Rachel's story is one that needs to be told because, in large measure, it is every NDD's story of the process; details differ, but the emotions are universal. Over 90,000 people are on the waitlist for a kidney donor, and until xenotransplantation becomes normalized or until people are financially motivated to become kidney donors, the vast majority of the people on that waitlist will die before they can get a transplant. It is through stories like Rachel's that we can educate people about the kidney crisis and the need for donors. I hope you enjoy Rachel's journey as much as I did.

*Ned Brooks*

Founder, National Kidney Donation Organization
(https://www.nkdo.org/)

Founder, Coalition to Modify NOTA (https://www.modifynota.org/)

# Prologue

As I walked along the five-mile route on Colorado Boulevard, bundled up in my long johns and brand-new sneakers, what struck me were the tears I saw in the eyes of the spectators. Those who brought their lawn chairs and blankets. Those who slept overnight together on the cold parkway as a family tradition. Those who were intentional about where they sat so they could have the best view of the parade as the floats passed by. I didn't cry until I saw them cry. It's a consequence of being an empath. Tell me how you feel, and I can't help but feel it too.

I didn't anticipate seeing so many tears in the sea of onlookers. After all, the Rose Parade is an exciting and magical experience, featuring colorful designs and ambitious marching bands, along with a sprinkling of famous people. But when your float celebrates life and memorializes those who became eye, organ, and tissue donors upon their deaths, something deep inside our core is triggered to respond. My path to be chosen to walk along the Donate Life Rose Parade float that year was nothing I ever envisioned for myself. Yet, it was always there; the alternate route.

For all the personality tests and quizzes that determine what kind of people we are, I can safely say that I am somewhere in the middle of most of them. By nature, I am an introvert. My comfort zone lies behind the scenes, where all the magic happens, allowing me to support those in the limelight as they do what they do best. If I had to choose between being the bride or the bridesmaid, I would be smoothing out wedding dress trains every day of the week. Here, let me hold your bouquet.

There have been certain circumstances where I have been one magical extrovert, however. When I am needed to be the voice, the face, or the vessel carrying the vital cargo, I can absolutely bring it home. When I look out into a crowd of people listening to what I have to say, that is when I am most uncomfortable, but I am also most impactful on the issues that I really care about. While I find peace and meaning in the shadows, my voice can illuminate an issue in ways that I hadn't fully appreciated until this adventure that I share with you now began to unfold.

How does an ordinary kind of person like me decide to do something that is deemed by the world community to be extraordinary? That is the million-dollar question university research departments have been studying for decades. If the "why" to altruism could be narrowed down, certainly more folks like me could be identified and encouraged to give of themselves. To donate one organ, or perhaps even more. Identifying those commonalities could prevent many people from needlessly dying while they wait for a miracle. Too many are waiting for a miracle in the form of a healthy but deceased organ donor.

Over the years, as I listened to and read about others who donated their kidneys to strangers, a common theme emerged in their explanations.

"It just made sense."

"It was the right thing to do."

"It was a no-brainer for me."

While I tend to agree with this sentiment, roses still need roots to bloom. A rose: its petals, its stem, and even its thorns do not magically appear one morning before sunrise. A rose gradually evolves from a seed into a blossom over time, through nature, and with nurture. The roots give it permission to grow and stretch toward the sky, nourishing the rose and allowing it to reach its full potential. All the activity happening under the surface, buried in the soil, collides to enable a bloom to even exist. Just as experience gives life to our decisions, roots give life to the rose.

It absolutely "makes sense" to donate an extra organ. Donation is "the right thing to do" for the good of humanity. However, if donating an organ were truly a "no-brainer," everyone would be doing it. There would be more of us existing in the world with one kidney. There would be less independent suffering and more collective compassion. That is the world I want to live in, where we look out for each other.

Over the long period of time that I reflected on my own donation road trip, I discovered a lot about myself and my own motivations for giving away my extra kidney. It was not a no-brainer for me. It took my entire brain to trigger this response. Years of justice work learned through the labor movement and my deeply ingrained working-class roots grounded me in this adventure. My family's connection to organ donation at an early age and the trauma my family has lived with since I was an infant also played a significant role.

Although my usually fleeting patience was put to the test, I successfully navigated the medical processes and appointments that were still being refined in the emerging world of kidney chains. This was not a quick process to bring to a conclusion at all, but the result, how my life evolved in the years after I woke up in the recovery room, was nothing I had ever imagined for myself. The community that awaited me on the other side and made my New Year's Day trek on Colorado Boulevard possible was unexpected yet absolutely necessary.

I am not implying that everyone who becomes an organ donor does so out of trauma, familial roots, or years of activism. It is more complicated than that. But it's certainly not as simple as it's "the right thing to do." After seeking answers within my own lived experiences about why I became a kidney donor, my story, like my kidney, needed to be shared.

Everyone has a story. Whether we decide to give of ourselves or keep all our gifts to ourselves, there will always be a backstory, even if we don't realize what it is at the time. Courage to do extraordinary things can be found within the stories we tell and the stories we hear. The courage to try. The courage to jump in the deep end. The courage to live another day. This is my story, with all its sadness, excitement, trauma, and humor. I invite you to join me in the deep end, friends, in whatever way you choose.

# Chapter 1

# Katie Couric Made Me Do It

*"Once you know something, you can't unknow it."*
*– Oprah Winfrey*

TV personalities have had a significant influence on my life. As a latchkey kid, I grew up with Oprah as my constant after-school companion. Through the stories of others, she taught me a lot about living purposefully and being a thoughtful person. Still today, I often find myself quoting something Oprah said so many years ago. "You only know what you know." "When you know better, you do better." "Listen to your inner voice." "You teach people how to treat you." Whether they were her own words or someone else's, I knew if Oprah said it, it was sound guidance to follow.

In my thirties, yet another prominent TV personality drew me in to stay informed by recapping the day's highlights. My work required me to be on the road across the country frequently, but whenever I was home on weekdays at 6:30 Eastern Time/5:30 Central Time, I tuned in to the *CBS Evening News with Katie Couric*. She was the first solo female anchor of a weekday network news broadcast and, as an advocate for representation, I happily supported her as a viewer. In fact, I owed it to her to sit on my couch and tune in—representation in all matters… matters.

The number of women doing the same work I did was minimal, given our representation in the manufacturing industry, which has been my workplace for most of my adult life. The very few women

I saw in leadership in my union convinced me that if I wanted to see more women in leadership, I had to support the women who were already there and be that leader myself. "Be the change you wish to see in the world." Didn't Oprah say that, too?

As an advocate and organizer for manufacturing and workers, I wasn't always concerned about who was doing what or how seeing women doing big things could transform our perceptions of society. That realization took decades of training and lived experiences. For me to meander from being a quiet night shift "shop-rat" to someone that has been affectionately or sarcastically referred to as a "community organizer" took a lot of investment that will never go unappreciated. Because gratitude runs deep, I owe the immense privileges I've had to all those who reached out a hand to me and led the way.

My relationship with Katie Couric was complicated because it was a one-way street. She didn't know someone in Middle America named Rachel was watching her show, or why I picked her. She fed me the news every night, and I digested it. The good, the bad, and the not-so-pretty were brought to me through those thirty minutes in front of the TV. I learned a great deal about the world and its people through her show. But it wasn't until she shared a story about a problem and a program which I knew nothing about that I realized she was talking directly to me. Maybe she knew I was watching after all?

"Every 90 minutes, someone dies waiting for an organ transplant."

Her first sentence of the segment held so much trauma. People are dying, folks. They are dying as they wait. Wait, why do they have to wait?

"Today, about 87,000 people are on the waiting list for a new kidney. But now a unique approach allowing donors and recipients to pay it forward is making more organs available."

"Kidney Chains Link Strangers" was the name of the news segment I was watching, in which Katie Couric reported.[1] A kidney chain had occurred the previous year, with ten people willing to donate their kidneys to ten strangers in need of a kidney. From New York to California, they all participated in this remarkable process that I had never heard of. A kidney chain *links* strangers. Very catchy.

It all started with an algorithm. In 2007, a New York couple, Jan and Garet Hil, experienced the frustration of trying to find a living kidney donor for their daughter, Samantha. The complicated matching process for donors and recipients put their search for a donor into a tailspin. Seven of their family members had been tested, and all of them were incompatible with Samantha. Eventually, the couple found a compatible donor for their daughter. Still, due to their own messy experience, they wanted to find a way to make the matching process between donors and recipients easier for others in similar situations.

Just like the Hil family, other families had people eager to donate a kidney to their loved ones, but were unable to because they were medically incompatible. The next best recourse for them was to identify someone else in the world who was compatible and ask them to donate. Finding two incompatible pairs of donors and recipients, who did not match the person they knew but matched the stranger, would allow for two transplants to occur that otherwise would not: Donor A gives to Recipient Z, in exchange Donor B gives to Recipient Y. Or even more broadly, Donor R gives to Recipient D and Donor O gives to Recipient Q, still without any of them knowing one another beforehand.

Hil, the CEO of a software company, and his team utilized their expertise to develop a sophisticated program that acted as a matchmaker, connecting incompatible pairs of potential donors and recipients with others who were also incompatible. The larger the pool of donors and recipients in the system, the more matches they could make and the more transplants they could facilitate.

Thus began the National Kidney Registry, and at the time of Katie Couric's news segment on November 10, 2010, it was the largest national database of living donors in the country. With 100,000 records specific to intended donors and recipients registered in the pool, an incompatible pair could match with other incompatible pairs somewhere else in the country in record time. The registry had the potential to create a chain reaction of donors and recipients, in a way never before considered, allowing more people to receive kidney transplants much more quickly.

Participating hospitals from across the country were pooling their donor and recipient data to find matches they could not find within their own, much smaller, isolated lists of candidates. It was a matchmaker's dream and an experiment in trust and cooperation for everyone relying on the registry to work its magic. But for any chain reactions to commence, someone had to kickstart the whole process, someone with a kidney to give, and no one in mind to receive it.

"It all started with this man, Max Zapata from Clovis, California, who kicked off this chain as the good Samaritan donor. He gave a kidney, expecting nothing in return."

The camera turned to Max Zapata, a middle-aged man with glasses and a big smile. He was sitting on an oversized brown sofa in a living room, flanked by smiling people, as he explained the rationale for his donation. He felt in his heart that he had to donate one of his kidneys. Max didn't know where it would go, but he knew he would be helping someone.

Katie Couric traced the kidney chain Zapata started through a series of clips and two-sentence interviews. Ten people were giving up their extra kidneys, and ten others were receiving those kidneys in total from across the country.

Zapata's kidney went to Laura, a 25-year-old college athlete. In exchange, her brother Paul gave his kidney to a 45-year-old geologist named Kirk. Kirk's wife, Teresa, donated her kidney to Melvin, an 83-year-old who was 3,000 miles away. Melvin's friend Tanya donated to Maria. In exchange, Maria's husband, John, donated to Simeon. Simeon's son, John, donated to Lee. In exchange, Lee's daughter, Lauren, donated to Daniel. Daniel's friend, Clint, donated to Fred. Fred's wife, Yvette, donated to Greg. Greg's Uncle Johnny was the last donor in the chain. His kidney went to Mindel, the last recipient. Mindel was expected to die until Uncle Johnny was discovered to be his perfect match.

Every donor in the chain was a stranger to the person who received their kidney. Because the software matched potential donors and recipients regardless of geography, the kidneys were much better matched as a result.

Aside from Max Zapata, the nine other donors — Paul, Teresa, Tanya, John, John, Lauren, Clint, Yvette, and Johnny — held the key to a better life for their spouses, friends, and family members. Donating a kidney to a stranger so that their loved ones could receive one from someone else in exchange is truly a gift. How can anyone ever top that at the next Christmas exchange? I could not imagine the admiration I would feel for someone in my family if they stepped up in this way for me, or anyone else, for that matter.

The segment ended with Zapata and some of the people from the kidney chain sitting around a long dinner table, bowed heads, as they said a prayer. Then they had a celebratory toast, with clinking glasses and adoring expressions. Couric concluded with the action call:

"If you'd like to learn how to be a part of a kidney chain, you can go to our website at cbsnews.com."

On that autumn night, Katie Couric spoke to the whisper that had been in my head for decades. I bet she had no idea how her news segment would impact viewers that day. Surely, I was not the only one who took her message and ran with it. I couldn't have been the only one who searched the internet for all the answers to all the questions, who told a friend, who tossed in the bed that night, wondering if there was a reason why she made me rethink what it meant to be kind. And that term "Pay it Forward." Yeah, I liked that.

I felt so intrigued and clueless that evening when I began my internet search and rescue mission.

What is the National Kidney Registry?

Where are my kidneys located?

What do kidneys do?

Before Katie Couric showed up in my living room with that story, I had little need to know anything about my internal organs. My health had never been a prominent factor in my life, aside from workplace injuries from years spent on the factory assembly line. Tendonitis, tennis elbow, cracked discs, and twisted fingers were the extent of my body telling me there were any issues. My kidneys never sounded any alarms. They worked fine, for all I knew.

The only information about kidneys that had been cemented in my brain came from my childhood, when I watched TV. It was a weekly ritual for Dad and me to watch WWF wrestling. *Superstars of Wrestling, Primetime Wrestling, Wrestling Challenge*; we watched them all. The announcers would frequently inform us when someone was getting tagged in the kidneys, which I speculated were located somewhere in their backs. Now, with this new news, I needed a better understanding of what was under the hood. I couldn't trust my memory of Rowdy Roddy Piper on this one.

Max Zapata had a look about him that caught my eye. I was intrigued to learn more about the kind of person who would give away an organ to a stranger, so I did some digging.[2] Zapata was a 50-year-old manager at a grocery store. It was not until he saw a public service announcement about organ donation at the bottom of his pay stub that he even thought about it. Once that seed had been planted, he was surrounded by signs, whispers in the back of his mind every day, until he finally decided to act on it. As a religious person, he credited his God for walking him along the path to start that kidney chain.

What stood out to me about Zapata was nothing and everything. He wasn't a triathlete or a finely tuned machine with an uber-active life. He wasn't an intellectual with a PhD in kidneys. He wasn't polished in any way that made me think he was out of my league. No bourgeoisie vibe was detected. If I walked past Max Zapata in a store or a movie theater, there would be no indication that he did this amazing thing for so many people he didn't even know.

Max Zapata was a member of the working class with limited means. He listened to his higher power and what he considered signs, and he acted upon them. He was a regular kind of guy who wanted to make a difference in the world in whatever way he could. The longer I thought about him, the more I was convinced: Max Zapata was just like me.

Coincidentally, *Kidney Chains Link Strangers* aired a few days before my birthday. Each year, I made it a habit to celebrate my birthday by doing something to express my gratitude to the world for giving me another year. My health and good fortune were cause for celebration in a way that was more about the bigger picture than about me. No spa day with the girlfriends or party in my honor was ever on the agenda. That is not who I am at my core. I am a quiet soul, a behind-the-scenes fixer of things, and a problem solver. I never wanted to be the star of any show, especially not on my birthday.

I had been doing this birthday regifting activity since my early twenties. It feels meaningful to do something outward each year, to be helpful to others. While my adoring partner, Mat, would occasionally throw me an awkward surprise party or celebrate with a fancy dinner, I do not have a fascination with celebrating *ME* on that day. The very fact that I am alive and well is reason enough to thank the stars for aligning each year.

My family was full of people with giving lives and caring hearts to learn from. Aunt Bev, Grana, and Dad; many bore the burden of compounding grief that needed to be channeled somewhere, and I regularly saw them doing good in their own ways. I would roll up my sleeve and donate blood with the Red Cross. Some years, I would attend a fundraiser for the St. Martin's free clinic in Garrett or the Workers Project in Fort Wayne. One year, I helped coordinate a garage sale with all proceeds going to the Relay for Life. Back then, I didn't have a specific passion or concrete focus in my gift-giving decisions, other than to be of use to someone, somewhere, somehow. What I was genuinely passionate about remained to be understood until long after Katie Couric first presented it to me in high definition.

In *Kidney Chains Link Strangers*, Garet Hil jokingly said, "I didn't even know I had two kidneys. That's how far off the radar it was," when he explained his path toward understanding the needs of his daughter. I, too, had no personal experience with kidneys to know anything about them. Kidneys were not my passion, but Katie Couric reaching into my living room that night in November rattled something in me. The idea of a kidney chain seemed like a highly effective way to help several people at once. I had not yet chosen what my birthday gift would be for that year, but I had something new to consider, thanks to the CBS Evening News with Katie Couric.

Max Zapata credited his faith in God for guiding him on his path to donate a kidney and start a chain that ultimately involved twenty people. It started with a message on his pay stub about organ donation. Then, kidney donation began to creep into his thoughts regularly, finally leading to his commitment. He listened to the whispers in his head, and twenty people are forever connected because of it.

My guiding light wasn't any particular God or spiritual being. I didn't discover my chosen faith community, Unitarian Universalism, until much later. For me, it was my grandmother. Grana had been vocal about organ donation since I was a kid. Her voice was quietly whispering in my ear as the kidney chain story unfolded on the news that night. Much like Oprah, she, too, was my voice of reason and goodness in the world. How to roll with all the punches life delivers without breaking a sweat is what I learned from Grana throughout my life. Months later, when I told her I was going to give away a kidney, I knew exactly how the conversation would conclude.

# Chapter 2

# **It Started with a Whisper**

The term "organ donation" was a common one I heard during my teenage years and into adulthood, as Grana often used it when talking about my Uncle Ed. My mother died by suicide when I was just an infant, so Grana played the role of the strong female lead throughout my life. She admirably became the nurturer-in-chief and the only person in my whole family to talk openly about everything all the time, even when it hurt, especially when it hurt.

Uncle Ed was the youngest of Grana's three children. Her other two children, my mother and her other brother, were quite a bit older than Uncle Ed, which put them in a position to care for him while Grana worked in food service. She never made more than $2.13 an hour plus tips, but managed to make ends meet with ingenuity and a hefty chunk of family teamwork. As is the case with single-parent families, the broader family unit must continually adapt and adjust.

My last memories of Uncle Ed are as a cool twenty-something-year-old uncle. He was tall. He lifted weights. He had a tanning-bed tan. He bought stuff for my sister, Dara, and me. He was a good uncle who invested time in us. As a kid, that was all that mattered. When a grown-up pays attention to you, well, that means you're certifiably special.

In the early years, we lived with our dad, three hours away in "The International City" of Lorain, Ohio. But every summer break from school, Dara and I would spend it with Grana in rural Indiana. On those lengthy annual vacations, we'd get passed around the family like mashed potatoes at the dinner table. Uncles, aunts, cousins, grandparents, great-grandparents; each of them taking a turn to give us some exposure to our matriarchal roots.

Uncle Ed's house had enough room in it to designate an entire room to his comic book collection. Maybe it's because I was so young, but that room felt huge with dozens of those white banker's boxes stacked to the ceiling. Each comic was tucked neatly into a plastic sleeve, numbered, and labeled.

Dara and I would sometimes go with Uncle Ed to the local comic bookstore. We'd stand next to him, barely able to see over the counter while he talked with the person standing behind it about "this" series or "that" original, which Uncle Ed already had in his possession. In that moment across the counter, he was a professional barterer, negotiating to swap one comic book for another to complete his most prized collections. Those whispered conversations felt so serious, like real risky business was taking place, and we were witnesses to it.

Rumor has it, Uncle Ed was sitting on a goldmine that would only appreciate over time like a fine wine or a wheel of Wisconsin cheddar. I wish I knew what his game plan was for his treasure. Did he plan on retiring early and living off the proceeds from Vintage First Edition Spiderman, or perhaps buy Grana a mansion, as you hear famous people do for their own mothers? In the end, I believe that room of organized wonder helped to pay for his funeral.

Northeast Indiana has been and remains a hub of manufacturing, from assembly lines to raw materials. Anyone who wanted to work with their hands was never short on options. Uncle Ed followed along in the family career path of making things. A local rubber mill hired him at an early age, as many of us living in the Midwest do. I don't recall him being happy with his job, but he always had money to spend on comic books and on us.

Uncle Ed not only worked hard at the mill, but he looked like he rolled around in it, too. It may not be immediately apparent, but working in a rubber mill means you are processing raw materials into rubber. Picture a large, antiquated industrial kitchen with various recipes, ovens, and mixing machines. If you plop your spatula into the flour bowl at home, a puff of white dust will rise and douse your face. Now imagine a rubber mill "kitchen" doing the same, except the puff of dust is as big as a cloud, is toxic, and is black.

Walking in the front door from his shift, he'd leave a trail of carbon black as he headed straight to the shower. His pile of dusty work clothes lived untouched in the corner until laundry day. There was always an excessive number of black Q-tips in the bathroom trash can. A white cotton swab was his tool of choice to remove the rubber recipe from the inside of his nose, his ears, and his eyes. The consequence of a working-class life is that you sometimes must do the least glamorous and most dangerous jobs around. Decades later, I'm proud to say it was my job to advocate for workers just like him to breathe a little easier.

We would have sleepovers at Uncle Ed's house and stay up late drinking pop, eating Cheetos, and watching movies. I remember us watching *Fast Times at Ridgemont High* there – no one took heed of movie ratings at the time. He took us to see E.T. at the local theater in town. We thought we were big time with hardly anyone else in the building. We had the theater all to ourselves. We had popcorn. Dara cried. I find my memory unusually clear on certain aspects of my life, which is bizarre given how young I was. I can't remember entire years of my childhood, yet Uncle Ed feels so prominent.

His extra motorcycle helmet was a little too big for us, but that didn't stop him from taking us along. My fingers wrapped around his belt loops as we rode down those country roads. And the burn mark I will forever have on my ankle from the exhaust pipe. The fact that I was too short to see what was ahead of us because he was blocking my view. These bits stay in my mind too.

Our first trip to Pokagon State Park was also with Uncle Ed during a winter break from school. The park had a toboggan run that, from the eyes of a child, looked like it began in the clouds. Neither Dara nor I had the winter gear necessary to weather the cold of a day playing outside, so he found the closest dollar store and bought our supplies: new hats, gloves, scarves, and snow pants.

He was a bachelor for a chunk of our childhood. Then, he met Yvonne, a nice lady from Van Wert, and the two of them hit it off. Dara and I were their junior bridesmaids when they married; I had a pink ribbon around my white dress, and Dara had a blue one. We continued to be permanent fixtures in both their lives, even after Uncle Ed's bachelor life became domesticated. Yvonne's younger brothers were close in age to us, so we all blended well into the family.

I know many people who bear the title of 'Uncle,' but too few take that responsibility personally and make an effort to be present in the lives of the children around them. It was a reflection of the love he felt for a sister gone too soon. He gave us that love and care in her absence. My Uncle Ed was "legit," as the kids say these days.

It would be naïve of me to think he was perfect, just because I knew him to be. He was a flawed human, just as we all are. He ate a lot of Kraft Macaroni and Cheese and drank too much Pepsi. He had a feisty side. He swore like a steelworker. He and Yvonne eventually parted ways, but not before my beautiful cousin Sam was conceived. Like my mother, he wrestled with his mental health regularly, without young people like me ever being the wiser.

Grana came to visit me and Dara to tell us when he died. It was important for her to do so in person because she knew how much we admired him. By then, I was 13, and Dara was 17. Dara cried while I stared silently at the floor, as I often did when Grana talked about the hard stuff. As kids, what else could we do?

I didn't grasp the details of his death back then or what it meant for our family. Grana said the police thought Uncle Ed's death might have been gang-related. Perhaps she wanted to believe that, which is why Dara and I never heard any other story about the cause of his death. It would take me decades to learn the truth and understand the interconnectedness of my family tree with my own origin story. My Uncle Ed lost the battle with his mental illness, dying by suicide.

The silver lining to Uncle Ed's death was that he became an organ donor. Grana and our family found something meaningful amid tragedy. I didn't know the term "organ donor" until Grana said it with such pride. Even as a kid, I knew it had to be something noble.

What happens when you lose a loved one is complicated. Immense grief and pain can overcome your senses, incapacitate you, and prevent you from seeing clearly. At a time when life-changing decisions need to be made, some may choose not to make any at all. The adults in our family, with Grana at the reins, decided to choose life instead of living with sorrow. Grana gave Uncle Ed's death the most positive swing imaginable: to save the lives of others.

As she and our family grieved our loss, Grana received mail that would become a permanent reminder of that decision for decades to come. Two letters were sent to let her know just how important Uncle Ed became to so many people across the country. The letter from Dr. Margaret Ball of the American Red Cross Tissue Services Department thanked Grana and described that Uncle Ed's tissue and bone donation would be used to treat burn patients and those in need of orthopedic bone repair. "It is possible for your son to help many people who await this specialized treatment," the letter explained.

Nurse Sandra Warner, a Procurement Coordinator with the Indiana Organ Procurement Organization (IOPO), sent a letter on behalf of them and Saint Joseph's Hospital in Fort Wayne, where Uncle Ed was pronounced dead. "Your love for your son became evident in the fact that you were willing to donate," she wrote. In the letter, Nurse Warner shared where Uncle Ed's organs went and who received them, with as much information as she was able to share without compromising anyone's privacy, of course.

In total, five people received Uncle Ed's organs. His heart went to a man who had been on the waiting list for quite some time. His liver went to a man from Indianapolis who was very sick. Uncle Ed's pancreas went to a man just a few years older than he was, which enabled him to stop taking insulin shots. Both of Uncle Ed's kidneys were transplanted. Because of his tissue typing, he was found to be a match for many. The lone female recipient of Uncle Ed's gifts had been waiting for six years for a new lease on life. She received one kidney. The other went to Puerto Rico, for a man who "will not need dialysis any longer," the letter shared.

I don't recall if Uncle Ed ever traveled the world. I'd guess he stayed close to home and let his exploration happen within the pages of his comic books. Still, knowing a piece of him was thriving on an island paradise that she herself never experienced must have made my Grana smile. There were no names or identifying markers to connect these recipients to real people. But knowing there were living, breathing humans on the other side of that trauma was a much-needed comfort.

My memory escapes me of when I first laid eyes on the letters. If Grana kept them close to herself at first, I don't recall. However, what I do remember from my childhood is that a copy of the letter from IOPO was in every room of her house. Because it gave Uncle Ed's death a deeper meaning, Grana never forgot about his donation or the letters, and she never wanted to.

Just three years after Uncle Ed's death, I faced my first question about organ donation head-on, at the Bureau of Motor Vehicles. The BMV is where most people are first asked the question:

"Do you want to register to become an organ donor?"

I was 16 when I got my driver's license. Unlike a lot of people that age, I had someone in my life who talked about organ donation often. Uncle Ed solidified my decision and the subsequent red heart proudly displayed on my Ohio driver's license.

When I graduated from high school, I moved from Ohio to Indiana. I knew I would have more opportunities in the neighboring state, having spent my summers there with Grana and our family. At 18, I moved into my Grana and her husband's basement and began the next phase of my life. As I became her housemate, I noticed a pattern in her emotional well-being, particularly during specific times of the year. The holidays, the summer, and Uncle Ed's birthday were hard for her. She was still mourning.

As she sat in that small tan rocker in the corner of the living room, she'd fumble through the junk drawer in the end table. It was one of many drawers in the house, filled with literal junk, but also contained nail polish, playing cards, phone books, and, of course, the letter. Grana would pull that letter from IOPO out of the drawer, look at it, and rock. She'd rock intentionally, as if she were putting her sorrows to sleep.

If I came into the room, she'd wave the letter at me. Then, she'd explain, as if for the first time, how many lives Uncle Ed saved. The letter became Grana's badge of honor. She was so proud of Uncle Ed, not only for his life but also for the way he helped so many after his death. She kept him alive in her mind through a simple but significant piece of paper.

As Grana aged and her focus began to blur, I became her quasi-caretaker and bill payer. I found the letters from the Red Cross and IOPO, still everywhere in her house. They were folded together in the desk drawer, the nightstand, and the kitchen junk drawer. I found a copy in her jewelry box that stood in the corner of her bedroom. She had boxes of pictures in her closet; the letter was there. And, of course, it was in the end table drawer next to her rocker.

I also have multiple copies of those letters now. I have a copy in my desk drawer, one in my safe, and one saved electronically on my computer. It's become a badge of honor for me and a reflection of the legacy I hope to carry on. A legacy of giving. A legacy of grit and tenacity. A legacy of rolling with the punches when you can't block them any other way.

When I told Grana I wanted to give away a kidney, she reacted as I expected her to. We were at the local Cracker Barrel eating breakfast together, as we did every Friday morning when I wasn't out of town. Sitting across from her on my third or fourth cup of coffee, I told her about Katie Couric and kidney chains and that I was signing up to give one away to a stranger. She asked if I would have to take pills after a surgery like that. When I told her no, that nothing would change for me after donating, she smiled, nodded, and replied, "Okay."

Then, she told me about Uncle Ed and his donation again, as if for the first time. And, like any grandkid worth their salt, I listened intently, as if for the first time.

Chapter 3

# Kidneys Are Kind of a Big Deal

In the days following my Katie Couric epiphany, I researched kidneys, kidney chains, and the National Kidney Registry. I was starting from scratch in this exploration, as I had no prior knowledge of the subject matter. I'd never let my naivete stop me from finding answers before. Investigative reporting and strategic sleuthing had become a way of life for me.

A big chunk of my twenties had been spent in college while working full-time building what most people would identify as "widgets and gadgets." Working third shift, which was in the middle of the night, and taking classes during the day or evening consumed my time. Auto parts and textbooks, production quotas and term papers; for many years, it all flowed together. Once I left the assembly line behind and began working for my union, the United Steelworkers, I continued to learn through the University of Massachusetts.

My program at UMASS Amherst required strategic research and in-depth analysis that was grueling but beneficial, not only for my work but for my ever-curious mind on all sorts of things. If I learned anything from my college experience, it was how to find credible answers to any question I had. Reading clinical trials, analyzing corporate financial data, and measuring environmental statistics had become an everyday occurence. College taught me how to paint the whole picture when contemplating an idea and to think critically about the world. But to be fair, so did my stint on the factory floor. There's no doubt about it.

Using all that know-how to understand kidneys and chains gave me a place to begin, with my initial questions about anatomy relatively easy to answer.

**Where are my kidneys and what do they do?**

My childhood observations from the World Wrestling Federation were correct; kidneys are situated in our backs. For most people, they press against our back muscles, right below our rib cage, on either side of the spine. The right kidney sits lower than the left one to make room for our liver, which sits above it. Kidneys can be slightly different in size, but are about the size of an adult clenched fist.

According to the National Kidney Foundation, kidneys are essential to the overall functions of our bodies. The primary responsibility of the kidneys is to sift waste out of the blood. They create urine by removing toxins and salt from the blood and regulating our fluid levels. It turns out, no matter how much water I drink, I'm not going to float away as I often heard growing up. Kidneys ensure that.

Kidneys also have the primary job of regulating blood pressure by releasing hormones that help control it and maintain red blood cell production. The kidneys regulate sodium, phosphorus, and potassium, and signal the body to produce Vitamin D, which helps maintain bone health.[3]

So yeah, kidneys are kind of a big deal. Imagine your body is a nightclub and your kidneys are the "bouncer." They enforce harmony and cohesion among all the things happening in the nightclub. Only the well-behaved can stay, and all the drunk or disorderly patrons get a swift kick in the arse. If there are too many patrons in the club, the bouncer kicks out the excess, all exiting through the same door, the urine stream.

**What happens to a kidney that requires a person to need a new one?**

Katie Couric opened her news segment with this staggering statistic.

"Today, about 87,000 people are on the waiting list for a new kidney. But now a unique approach allowing donors and recipients to pay it forward is making more organs available."

With kidneys having so many important jobs in the body, and so many people needing a new one, how and why kidneys fail sounded like an epidemic.

A lot can happen to a kidney that compromises its ability to do its job, primarily falling under the umbrella term "kidney disease." When kidneys are damaged and unable to filter blood properly, they can fail. High blood pressure and diabetes pose the most significant risk for developing kidney disease.[4] Both can damage the blood vessels in the kidneys to the point of disrepair.

Genetic conditions and abnormal development also cause failure. The list of conditions is extensive, and their technical terms are equally complex. Things like Polycystic Kidney Disease (PKD), Berger's Disease, and posterior urethral valves can affect the kidneys, to name just a few.

An emergency back-up to non-functioning kidneys is dialysis. If the kidneys can't filter waste from the body, a dialysis machine can do it for them. It looks like the machine used at the Red Cross to collect blood platelets for donation, but with one major difference. A dialysis machine pulls blood out, cleans it of toxins, and then returns the good stuff. For many, dialysis gets them by until they can find a donor and receive a transplant. But for some, dialysis becomes their way of life and their only option. Dialysis becomes a part of their new normal.

The waitlist Katie Couric referred to is where the names of people in need of a kidney, heart, lungs, liver, pancreas, or small intestine transplant are kept until a match from a deceased donor is found. The list, coordinated by the United Network for Organ Sharing (UNOS), comprises individuals from across the country who require one or more of these organs to save their lives. Finding a donor organ match can take decades, and everyone on the list must wait their turn in the invisible but growing line.[5]

Waiting for someone to die so an organ becomes available sums up the agony of this list. Waiting for the death of a donor like my Uncle Ed so that another may live is neither a tragedy nor a gift; it's both. As people who are waiting receive their transplants, they are removed from this list. Those who die waiting, about thirteen people every day, are also removed from the list. Then, those waiting behind them move up in line. Uncle Ed's organs saved the lives of five people from Indiana to Puerto Rico, which allowed five others to move closer to the top of the list to their lifesaving moment.

As our loved ones pass away and become donors, the waitlist should decrease. But as the supply of donated organs increases, so does the demand. According to Donate Life America, someone new is added to the list every eight minutes.[6] Our population is becoming sicker, in more ways than one.

In 2010, when Katie Couric aired her segment on kidney chains, the transplant waitlist had 87,000 people in need of a kidney. Sixteen years later, in 2026, more than 94,000 people are on that same list, waiting for that same organ.[7] More people need kidneys than there are deceased donor kidneys available. Something must be done. Enter living donors…

**What kind of living, breathing people give away their organs?**

Living kidney donation has become an alternative for many people waiting for a deceased donor kidney. It gives very sick folks a second option at a healthy new start. The first successful living kidney transplant happened in 1954 between Richard and Ronald, the Herrick twins.[8] Since then, living donors have had a small, yet constant presence, often inconspicuous, in the world of transplantation.

Organ Procurement and Transplantation Network (OPTN) data show that there were 194,727 living kidney donors from 1988 through the end of 2025, of whom 112,655 were blood relatives of the recipient.[9] A parent donating to a child, a sibling giving to a sibling, a child giving to their grandparent. You get the drift. Friends, spouses, and partners donating kidneys have helped fill the remaining gap in donors.

Tucked into the data is a very small but mighty row of numbers titled "Non-Biological Unrelated Anonymous Donors.[10]" The Max Zapatas of the nation are tracked annually in this data set. In the years preceding 2010, when I conducted my search, non-directed donors seemed like unicorns. In 2006, a mere 68 people donated a kidney to someone they didn't know. In 2007, that small number was 97 people, and in 2008, only 106 people donated to a stranger. That number increased in 2009 to 134, but it was still a relatively insignificant number when looking at the whole picture of living donors. There were millions of Americans walking around with an extra ticket to life, but only enough Max Zapatas existed to fill five school buses.

Even though 515 more non-directed donors were added to the count in 2025, they still seem like unicorns.[11] With just 5,983 of them on record since 1988, all of the non-directed, non-biological, unrelated, anonymous donors from the last 30 years could fit on the same cruise ship together, with plenty of room for a conga line and a live band. Meanwhile, the 94,187 folks who need a kidney would have the Rose Bowl stadium bursting at the seams, with a line out the door.

Donation between people who know each other makes a lot of sense. If you see your friend or child enduring years of pain and suffering, the urge to help is instinctual. Years ago, Mat had a good friend, Parker, with a terminal brain tumor who needed blood donations. By all accounts, Parker was the life of the party in our twenties and full of piss and vinegar. Many people in our community stepped up to help, including some who had never donated before. Of all the times we donated blood through the years, that was the only time I ever knew where it went. It felt like a more urgent commitment than at any other time we rolled up our sleeves, because he was important to us.

Being a non-directed kidney donor requires a belief that other people, even those we don't know, are also important to us. People who are strangers, unknown, or may never be known, who are out there struggling in the world, are embraced in this peculiar community as one of their own. The notion that we should be looking out for each other, in whatever way we can, is the non-directed donor's creed. It's also the philosophy behind deceased donation. Uncle Ed's organs went to whoever needed them the most at the time, no matter who they were. For some, embracing the broader world as our own means giving away body parts to save the lives of those unmet.

**Is the National Kidney Registry (NKR) leading the charge?**

Information about kidney chains available in 2010 was concentrated in just a few resources. Since NKR was in its second year of operation, there wasn't a wealth of knowledge to draw from about the organization. I searched for financial data and IRS Form 990s to no avail. I wasn't looking for dirt, but rather just any information I could find.

NKR was based in New York, with just a few members of the leadership team listed on the website. In his staff picture, Garet Hil bore a resemblance to the familiar face of an actor-turned-action hero from the past: David Hasselhoff. I remember, as a kid, watching Michael Knight and Kit fight crime as Dad and I ate potato chips on the couch. I wonder how many times Garet had been mistaken for someone's childhood memory.

As I scrolled through the website and read the frequently asked questions, NKR appeared to have it together. I was pleased and surprised at its very laid-back, non-aggressive appeal to living donors. The website didn't portray a desperate plea for my kidney, but if I wanted to donate, NKR could help. For me, what it lacked in organizational history, NKR made up for in its mission and its moment in the spotlight with Katie Couric.

The media page, with articles and features from newspapers and TV, transported me across the country, into the lives of those who had already given their kidneys away to strangers.[12] Personal testimonies of this kind, where individuals are interviewed in their homes about the impact of kidney donation on them as both donors and recipients, are the best marketing tool one could have. I absorbed all that I could find, seeking inspiration and understanding.

On Valentine's Day, 2008, 50-year-old California native Cindy Marshall donated one of her kidneys to a man in New York, causing a chain reaction for eight other surgeries among strangers.[13] Dr. Sandip Kapur, the transplant program director at New York Presbyterian Hospital, where most of the surgeries took place, said, "An altruistic donor unlocks the key to the whole process. This is an innovative system to keep people alive."

As a former Marine, Marshall's decision to start a chain was influenced by her family. Her husband donated his kidney to his brother twelve years prior, and witnessing how well he did after surgery was motivating to her. At the same time, Marshall watched a TV program highlighting the evolving positive perception of non-directed donation, as surgery techniques became less invasive and grueling. It gave her the courage to reach out to NKR.[14]

On December 2, 2008, the second-longest kidney chain, and the longest ever started by a woman, began.[15] Christina Do, a 36-year-old real estate investor, initiated a chain of donations involving 11 donors and 11 recipients, all of whom were scattered across four New York City hospitals. It was a combination of reading about kidney patients and the effects of the recession on the country that convinced Do to become a donor.

"So many people were upset about losing money," she says, "but what I got out of the recession was that there are more important things than money. It made me think about what kind of person I really wanted to be. And I decided I wanted to really help someone."

Do was able to meet some of the people in the chain a year after their surgeries. Even though she was content with never knowing any of them personally, it reinforced her decision to see that they were all doing well.

In March of 2009, a 12-person kidney chain was initiated between three hospitals in New York and New Jersey over 36 hours.[16] The three-part series featured by *The Star Ledger* read like a suspense novel, full of anticipation and anxiety, hope and fear, love and, of course, pain:

"Key to the process was a hero, known to doctors and nurses simply as a non-directed donor." The rarest of medical anomalies, these people are willing to give up a perfectly good kidney for altruistic purposes alone – not to help a friend or relative, but to help create a chain and make it happen. They are the quintessential good Samaritans."

Tom Leger, a 27-year-old writer, teacher, and businessman, was the good Samaritan donor who started this chain. He was guided by an article he read about philanthropy and the obligations of the rich, titled "What Should a Billionaire Give – and What Should You?" by Peter Singer. In it, Singer told of a wealthy man who gave away most of his fortune and one of his kidneys because he believed it was the right thing to do. Leger agreed.

Leger also had personal reflections that convinced him to donate: his own body. As a transgender man, Leger was able to affirm his true self, and wanted to help others who were facing physical and medical challenges they could not solve alone. Donating a kidney was his way to help.

In the spring of 2010, Loyola University Medical Center in Chicago started the first kidney chain to originate in Illinois. Christina Lamb, a 45-year-old from Melrose Park, wanted to donate years earlier to her husband, but was not a match. Because she witnessed her husband's progress and improved quality of life once he received a kidney from his cousin, she wanted to give that gift to someone else through donation. "Someone close to us gave my husband the gift of life; I felt it was important to do the same," she said.[17]

Three donors and three recipients from Illinois, Indiana, and Missouri were a part of this historic first for the state. When asked why he didn't keep the kidney chain among his own patients rather than sharing it with the best match across the region, the director of the Loyola program, Dr. John Milner, said, "We see every good Samaritan donor as a national treasure, not an institutional commodity."

A national treasure.

Much like the Katie Couric news segment, Loyola also used the term "pay it forward" to describe its program. Catchy and oh so true.

The term "pay it forward" transports me to the Wendy's drive-thru during the holiday season. My sister, Dara, was good at surprising the car behind her in the drive-thru by paying for their food before they even reached the window. Imagine, one minute you're anxiously awaiting your frosty and large fries, and the next you're feeling all warm and fuzzy over somebody you only know by the size of their bumper. Dara began doing that holiday goodwill gesture because someone did the same thing for her once, creating a chain reaction of paying it forward, one cup of chili at a time.

There were more than a dozen articles and news segments similar to these posted on the website and on local news websites. The donors were just like Max Zapata, who was called to step forward out of a sense of service and a whisper. A whisper that was getting louder after reading an article, after watching a news segment, after seeing a loved one bounce back after a transplant. Those who received kidneys in these exchanges looked forward to returning to work, to building that back porch, to finishing that college degree that was put on hold because of a debilitating disease. The motivation, nestled in their personal dreams and goals, kept them alive until a kidney came to the rescue. But not everyone is as fortunate.

Kidney failure not only weighed on the hearts and minds of those who lived with it, but it also weighed on their finances. Kidney disease is expensive.

Chapter 4

# Kidney Donation is Economic Justice

In the publications tab on the National Kidney Registry website, a report from 2009 was featured with the title: "Kidney Transplants Facilitated by a National Registry Can Save $100 Billion in U.S. Healthcare Costs.[18]" The white paper was NKR's appeal to Washington, D.C., lawmakers to see the bigger kidney picture. Not only could a national registry like theirs save and improve more lives, but it could also save money.

While private insurers provided coverage for one-third of all people undergoing dialysis or receiving a transplant, Medicare picked up the tab for the rest. The most significant expense for insurers was the cost of dialysis treatments, which, at the time, averaged $51,000 per patient annually. When medications, therapies, and other related medical expenses are added, the annual cost of care for all patients with end-stage renal disease (ESRD) reaches $30 billion.

The report argued that increasing the number of transplants each year would reduce the financial burden on Medicare and private insurers. With kidney transplant aftercare costing less than $9,000 per recipient per year, the math spoke for itself, even with the cost of the transplant factored in. If you had a choice to spend $51,000 to get by or $9,000 for a new lease on life, which would you choose? But was it that easy?

Given the already overburdened wait list, where more people are waiting for a deceased donor kidney than would ever become available, the only way this cost-saving plan could be realized was to presume that living donors would lead the charge and pick up the remaining slack. They were indeed the secret recipe in this equation to save the government and private insurers even more money.

Kidneys transplanted from living donors last, on average, eighteen years, while those from deceased donors have an average lifespan of ten years. With NKR's ability to provide the best possible match between a donor and a potential recipient, a living donor kidney could potentially last even longer, thereby alleviating the need for a recipient to undergo a second or third transplant later in life. The more living donors there are, the better the matches, resulting in significant cost savings.

I knew the report was designed to appeal to policymakers or academics, but it also put a price on the concept of freedom, and that resonated with me.

At the time, my dad worked for the county council on aging. He and a few other staff members drove the minivans and short transit buses that transported DeKalb County residents of all ages to where they needed to go. Each Tuesday afternoon, he would pick up the ladies from the senior apartment complex and drive them to their weekly lunch spot. Then Dad would pick them up later for their trip to buy groceries. He'd take kids from school to their latch-key programs. He'd take elders from the nursing home to their holiday dinners with family. Each day promised a variety of destinations with assorted patrons, leading him down various country roads in all kinds of weather.

But the one trip he made regularly, every day, with multiple riders, was to the dialysis center. For a town with fewer than 13,000 people, Auburn had two of these centers. Being the county seat, they provided services to the entire county of 42,000 people. Dad was a regular at both centers, dropping off riders in the early hours of the day and then, after several hours, picking them up.

He didn't tell me details about his passengers, but I know it weighed on him to see so many people in tow for the same reason. Neither of us has been formally declared empathetic[19], but feeling what other people feel sits heavily on one's shoulders, I can attest. To absorb that in the daily grind of your workplace, on the road, had to be tough for him. In 2009, there were nearly 400,000 people across the country, like those riding in the minivan with Dad. And each year thereafter, 100,000 more were predicted to be added to the dialysis ranks.[20]

I don't mean to be a "dialysis downer." Dialysis does what the kidneys can no longer do. It filters toxins from the blood, regulates the amount of fluid carried, and allows people to sustain themselves for the rest of their lives, or as long as necessary, until they receive a transplant. It is life-sustaining. But at the same time, it's a life-commitment.

The average treatment time required for a dialysis patient is equivalent to a part-time job. The body needs to be cleansed of its toxins for an average of 3 days a week, for 4 hours each day, to sustain itself.[21] Considering the investment of time and energy a process like this requires, it is enough to put even the most determined person out of work and out of hope. There are also options for those needing dialysis to perform this process at home on their own, but it requires a lot of skill and care. Supplies and machine parts can accumulate throughout the house, with cords and hoses often tangled in the corners. Many dialysis patients do not choose that route.

Spending half the day hooked up to a machine, either at a dialysis center or at home, diminishes one's ability to participate in gainful employment, if it's possible at all. Sure, there are occupations with flexible work schedules and accommodating bosses, but how can anyone concentrate on paying the rent when fluid levels and dialysis appointments are looming over their head? And how does one hold onto hope with all that rigmarole further complicating their lives?

At the time I was considering donating, I was a field coordinator for the Alliance for American Manufacturing, a manufacturing advocacy group. For me, "the field" spanned nine different states and the District of Columbia. I drove or flew to various parts of the country every week to conduct my work. My days were long, often lasting 10 to 12 hours of face-to-face interaction, during which I had to be on my game. I could not imagine pretending to feel well and fully focused on the task at hand if I were someone with kidney disease. Plus, needing to always have a dialysis center nearby would have been unrealistic.

But a dialysis patient isn't the only one who bears a burden. Spouses and family members help pick up the slack financially and domestically because they want to alleviate the suffering of their loved ones. Imagine planning a family vacation based on the location of the closest dialysis center and then feeling sick and bloated while sitting on that roller coaster with your child. Or, you need to stay back in the hotel room to recover and rest while they explore the Grand Canyon without you. Missing the choir recital because it interferes with dialysis, or your cousin's wedding, because it's just too far away.

Those in the back seat of Dad's minivan were all missing out on living because they were spending so much time trying not to die. Dialysis was costing them so much more than their copays and deductibles. It was costing them their freedom, too.

**So, a kidney transplant must cost a zillion dollars, right?**

According to the Milliman Report, which estimated average transplant costs for 2008, the average cost of a kidney transplant was $260,000, with Medicare and private insurance covering the bulk of the expense. That number reflected the total cost, not simply the cost of inserting a kidney into someone who needed it.

Consider the whole package: 30 days of care before the transplant, procurement, hospital admission, a transplant surgeon, 80 days of post-operative care, and 180 days of medication. Honestly, that sounded like a steal to me; to receive a fully functioning organ that offered newfound freedom and health for less than the cost of a mortgage.

I looked at this dollar figure from a "Rate-of-Return" point of view. Considering that one year of dialysis costs approximately $51,000, it would take slightly more than five years to break even. With the cost of maintenance medication and follow-up care being $9,000 each year, a transplant recipient could leave the machine behind and make that drive to their cousin's wedding after all. Dad would have had fewer people in the minivan to transport across the county for dialysis, but that'd be alright with him.

Tucked into the figures of the Milliman Report were costs associated with getting the appropriate kidney to a recipient, also known as "procurement." According to the 2008 report, this line item totaled $67,500. Frighteningly, that was much more than my annual salary, which begged the question:

**How much could it cost *ME to give a kidney away?***

The NKR website briefly outlined the donation process and provided considerations for potential donors. For starters, all associated costs of removing a kidney for transplant would be absorbed by the recipient of the kidney. Because organ procurement from a deceased or living donor was a necessary part of the process, it was covered by both Medicare and private insurers. The show could not go on without someone like my Uncle Ed or me; hence, we both got into the club for free.

Knowing there wasn't a medical financial burden made this a more appealing proposition. It may be evident by now, but Mat and I have never been rich in the green stuff. With roots firmly planted in the working class, we've never aspired to be interviewed by Robin Leach on *Lifestyles of the Rich and Famous*. I still remember that day in 1995 when I was wealthy enough to choose the box of Tide detergent at Kroger instead of the Purex. With solid financial advice from my Grana, we managed to eat multiple times a day while simultaneously staying off the cover of the *Forbes* "Richest People in the World" issue. Our motto had always been "live like you're broke so you never will be." It's in this frugal life code that we invest our energy to live free from the influence of the Joneses.

While transplant savings and expenses were essential to calculate, the overarching effect of money on the well-being of our most vulnerable spoke to the core values I held. My experiences with employers led me to the conclusion that decisions were almost exclusively made by weighing financial costs, without a second thought for equity. To me, if money, or the saving of it, could lead to freedom, then donating an organ could help balance the scales of justice.

I had been a member of the Steelworkers union since I was 18, when I got my first full-time job in an automotive factory. Quite a few members of my extended family were in unions, but I had never been in a union hall, on a picket line, or even heard them "talk shop" during my childhood. As a new adult, I had to maneuver through not only a new job but also union work rules. And, damn, were there rules.

As the years passed, I came to appreciate how important those rules and the union contract were to my coworkers and me. It prevented employer abuse and clarified, in writing, the pay and working conditions for everyone in the factory. Under that contract, we were protected from discrimination, pay disparity, and favoritism. Looking out for one another was the central premise of our union's existence, with justice at its core.

My activism in the union grew beyond my own factory as I helped other workers secure their own union contracts or campaign to keep their workplaces open. I undertook research projects for our district office aimed at increasing wages for some of the most marginalized workers in our region. Eventually, I worked for our international union office, assisting small workplaces and entire industry groups alike in bargaining improved contracts with their employers, thereby securing better pay and benefits for their families.

As a field coordinator, advocating for domestic manufacturing jobs, fair trade policies, and infrastructure investment, my work centered around creating good jobs with pay and benefits that supported working families. It was my responsibility to seek justice for workers who had been unemployed and unfairly affected by poor public policy decisions and, even worse, by unfair trade agreements.

In union halls and universities, I taught what I had learned; we must look out for each other in every way we can. The notion of solidarity, that mutual support was our primary obligation to each other, had become embedded in the way I lived my life. The bigger picture, which I was trained to see in all its ambiguities, convinced me that justice took many forms along the way, but would always be the ultimate goal.

As I deliberated on the financial aspects of this newfound version of solidarity, I felt a sense of fellowship with those in need of a transplant. I didn't know anyone in search of a kidney, yet their lack of freedom and the helplessness that must go along with it filled me with sadness. Usually, when I think about economic justice work, it's a minimum wage law, a tax policy, or a housing credit that comes to mind. However, returning to an everyday life, earning a living, and taking care of one's family is also a form of economic justice. In this scenario, it is only possible if others step forward with a gift greater than cash.

In philosopher Peter Singer's article "What Should a Billionaire Give – and What Should You?[22]" he poses the question:

"What is a human life worth?"

As a leading voice on the study of effective altruism, Singer analyzed the philanthropic work of Bill and Melinda Gates and Warren Buffett, wondering if they, despite giving billions away to alleviate global poverty, had done enough. The Gates' financial commitment to eradicating diseases in the developing world brought them high praise around the globe and credit for saving the lives of millions of children. But did this enormous haul allow them to sleep well at night if they were still living in a mansion? Are the Gates and others required to still give more because they still have more?

Singer pointed to Zell Kravinsky, a successful 40-year-old real estate investor. He kept his modest home and enough money to pay his regular family expenses, then gave away his entire fortune, almost $45 million, to charity. But he didn't stop there.

Once he learned of the need for living kidney donors, Kravinsky gave away one of his kidneys to a stranger. For him, given the slim risks associated with donation, valuing his own life more than that of a person in need seemed illogical. Despite his wife's objections and the fact that he had young children who might eventually need his kidney, Kravinsky chose to see the stranger as an equally valued person in need of saving.

Fortune, however big or small, was at the heart of the matter. When we consider our own personal giving, do we think all human lives have equal value, and if so, is that belief reflected in our actions? I understood why Tom Leger was inspired by Peter Singer's New York Times article enough to give his own kidney away and start a chain. And if we truly consider it, we can do so much more to help those in need than we already do. What if the rich and the not-so-rich would give more than just money? What if we saw our fortune as more than just our bank account balance?

**Transplant Costs with each Milliman Research Report:**

2008: Total: $259,000, of which $67,500 was for procurement[23]

2011: Total: $262,900, of which $67,200 was for procurement[24]

2014: Total: $334,300, of which $84,400 was for procurement[25]

2017: Total: $414,800, of which $96,800 was for procurement[26]

2020: Total: $442,500, of which $113,900 was for procurement[27]

2025: Total: $446,800, of which $135,400 was for procurement[28]

# Chapter 5

# Can I Get My Kidney Back?

To dig a little deeper into the technical and physical side of donation, I looked to a very useful "Myths about Living Donation" guide featured on the NKR website[29]. Each myth presented in the guide was countered with guidance, research, and statistics, helping quickly address many reservations one might have about life after donating a kidney. It was authored by Marian Charlton, a nurse, and Ilana Silver Levine, a social worker, so I felt assured that they were knowledgeable about the subject. The guide explained many things that were curiosities for me, but reading through them also made me doubt how qualified I was to be a donor in the first place.

*Myth #1: A kidney donor will take medications for the rest of their life.*

*Fact #1: A kidney donor is given prescriptions for pain medication and stool softeners at discharge from the hospital. These are only for the immediate post-operative period. After that time, the donor will no longer need to take medication.*

*For me*, this myth most likely arose because kidney transplant recipients need to take medication their whole lives for their body to accept a new organ. Without this medicine, the body would presume the kidney is an intruder and attack it with its own immune defenses. Anti-rejection medicine essentially takes away the immune system's ability to fight off the new organ. The downside is that the medicine also prevents the recipient from fighting off diseases and infections. There is no reason for donors to take lifelong medications because nothing new is introduced into the body to maintain or safeguard, as recipients must do.

*Myth #2*: *A kidney donor will have debilitating pain for an extended period of time.*

*Fact #2*: *A kidney donor has some pain after surgery from both the incisions and related to gas and bloating. This pain diminishes in the days following surgery and is controlled with pain medication if necessary.*

*For me,* I worked in a very physical occupation for well over a decade. I ran assembly lines that applied adhesives to metals for the automotive industry. The parts varied in shape and weight, but required me to adapt as necessary. In those years on the shop floor, I had a myriad of workplace injuries from tendonitis to cracked discs in my spine. I knew all too well what "debilitating pain for an extended period of time" felt like. Removing a kidney would be far from that sort of pain.

*Myth #3:* *A kidney donor will be on bed rest following surgery.*

*Fact #3:* *A kidney donor will be out of bed and walking independently before discharge from the hospital.*

*For me,* I guessed this surgery would be intense, with some pain and discomfort. Catheters would be involved, along with IVs, saltine crackers, and flat 7-Up. To remove an organ meant that at least one incision would need to be made, considering a kidney is the size of a fist. Plus, kidneys are attached to other things that would need to be patched up, with hoses sealed and tubes tied. A wild water hose flailing around with urine pouring throughout my innards was my first image of the moments after my kidney would be disconnected from me. There is no internal valve to shut off the flow. In actuality, medical-grade clips are used, much like an industrial banding machine.

*Myth #4:* *A kidney donor is in the hospital for an extended period of time after surgery.*

*Fact #4:* *A kidney donor is hospitalized for two nights.*

***For me,*** I had never been hospitalized in my life. All the procedures and doctor's visits I have ever had were outpatient. Even when I cracked two discs and needed surgery, it was an outpatient procedure, and I walked out of the building that very same day. I wasn't nervous or scared of being hospitalized; I just didn't have any experience with it. Perhaps the staff would tuck me in and keep a watchful eye for the two days of my luxurious stay? Room service? Chocolates on the pillow? That would be alright with me.

Given that kidney donation was considered a major surgery, the time needed to recover was of concern to me, however. My work-life would need to be factored in, and advanced planning would be necessary. Meetings and events could be rearranged or done remotely, provided I had notice to make it happen. I naively envisioned December, the very next month, for this surgery to happen. It was usually a slow month for my work assignments, and it seemed like the most logical month to be hospitalized, with plenty of time to recover through the holidays.

***Myth #5:*** *A kidney donor can no longer participate in sports or exercise.*

***Fact #5:*** *A kidney donor can return to regular activities and exercise at approximately 4-6 weeks following surgery.*

***For me,*** I have never been personally invested in sports. The closest I ever came to athleticism was the Monday night bowling league for the factory. Mat and I played on a team called "The Strikers" or something similarly catchy. We bowled for fun, not for blood.

I did exercise, though, enough to invest in a gym membership for the times the roads were covered in snow. I was a walker and a bike rider. I did yoga and lifted weights. Kickboxing was my most aggressive exercise of choice, but I rarely practiced it with another person. Bob, the Body Opponent Bag, was my sparring partner, and he never hit back.

***Myth #6:*** *A kidney donor has to follow a new diet plan following donation.*

***Fact #6:*** *A kidney donor should eat a healthy, well-balanced diet. There are no dietary restrictions following donation.*

***For me,*** given my history, I honestly wasn't convinced I was healthy enough to donate in the first place. Sure, the Max Zapatas of the world were healthy enough to donate, but did they survive on canned ravioli and Hamburger Helper throughout their childhoods? As an adult, I have eaten much better since I could afford to, but all that processed food from dinners past had to factor into this somehow, right?

Growing up in Lorain, Ohio, I lived near several steel mills, with the steady stream of smokestacks signaling prosperous times. Lake Erie, where "Do Not Swim, Water is Contaminated" signs dotted the beaches, bordered my city to the north, and was a regular spot for our family to visit. Sure, Lorain was known for much more than its air and water pollution. It was home to Toni Morrison, one of the most celebrated authors in the world, for crying out loud! But for my kidneys, how did my internal composition endure that sort of environmental beating? I wasn't so concerned with my eating habits now or after a kidney donation. I was concerned that my past could throw a wrench into the whole idea.

***Myth #7:*** *A kidney donor can no longer consume alcohol following donation.*

***Fact #7:*** *While excessive alcohol use is always dangerous, a kidney donor can consume alcohol in moderation.*

***For me,*** as an adult, I enjoy a good craft beer or a glass of wine every now and then. I am a bit of a lightweight, really, feeling loopy after just one. Since I hadn't already become an excessive drinker due to exposure to alcoholism from those around me, the likelihood of my becoming one after a kidney donation was slim.

My drinking days had come and gone as I was a regular beer drinker during my teenage years. Long before it became a cannabis-infused drink, forties (40 oz.) of everybody's favorite malt liquor, St. Ides, were common in my circles on a weekend. And before you clutch the pearls, know this: young, impressionable people do what the people around them do. My friends and our boyfriends all drank and smoked weed. We smoked weed before it was taxable, before it was a lucrative, progressive business venture.

I had a lot of drinkers and chain smokers in my family in the early years. People who drank and smoked all day, every day, and this was before anyone gave secondhand smoke a second thought, not to mention third-hand smoke. I still remember getting out of the car as a kid, in a cloud of smoke. Like a music video where the dancers were surrounded by fog for the effect, except this wasn't fog, and I wasn't dancing.

My decade in the factory required me to ingest toxins regularly. I worked in the paint room with industrial coatings that smelled of rubber cement. Our exhaust system did its best to filter the danger out of the air, but the ceilings in the department were low, and there's only so much protection one could be assured of in such an environment. Exposure to all of these things weighed on my mind as I maneuvered through the information. My innards were probably barely holding it together by now. Was I wasting my time?

*Myth #8: A female kidney donor should not get pregnant after donation.*

*Fact #8: A female kidney donor should wait 3-6 months after donation to become pregnant. The body requires time to recover from the surgery and to adjust to living with one kidney before pregnancy.*

*For me,* Mat and I decided long ago, as our siblings provided ample quantities of offspring for our family lineage, that we had no obligation to join them. In 2010, I had close to twenty kids who lovingly called me Aunt Rae. Many were our nieces or nephews through marriage or genes, while others were the children of close friends who latched on.

We have always had a fondness for children. They are fun, and each one is unique, like a snowflake or a potato salad recipe. Yes, they are indeed great, especially when they're somebody else's, when you can give them back to their parents, then have your freedom to do as you please. That was the life we purposefully chose, so pregnancy questions related to kidney donation were of no concern to me.

*Myth #9: A kidney donor's sex life is negatively affected by donation.*

*Fact #9: A kidney donor may engage in sexual activity whenever they feel well enough to do so.*

*For me,* did I miss that day of anatomy class? To clarify, your kidneys are located on either side of your spine, positioned just below your rib cage. This is nowhere near your sex parts.

The long-term health effects for someone living without a backup kidney were also crucial for me to know. I did not want to increase my personal risk of my lone kidney failing later in life and having to endure the same dialysis regimen that the folks I wanted to help were currently experiencing. Fortunately, several studies addressed my concern.

In Sweden, 430 kidney donors who donated between 1964 and 1994 were evaluated to assess their health over a 20-year span.[30] The authors found that donors' health and mortality were the same or better than those of the general population.

Its conclusion: "To donate a kidney does not seem to constitute any long-term risk. The better survival among donors is probably due to the fact that only healthy persons are accepted for living kidney donation."

Cleveland Clinic studied 70 of its donors over 25 years, from 1963 to 1975, to evaluate their kidney health.[31]

Its conclusion: "Overall, renal function is well preserved with a mean follow-up of 25 years after donor nephrectomy. Males had significantly higher protein and albumin excretion than females. Still, no other clinically significant differences in renal function, blood pressure, or proteinuria were noted between them or at the age of donation."

In Tokyo, a study of 1,519 people who donated from 1971 to 2007 was conducted to understand risk factors for end-stage renal disease.[32] Eight of those in the study developed kidney disease later in life. They tracked all eight donors by evaluating their medical files to understand how and when kidney disease became prevalent. Cardiovascular issues, diabetes, smoking, car crashes, and protein in the urine were factors in their health after donation.

Its conclusion: "They do not necessarily have chronic kidney disease (CKD) risk factors before donation, but they develop these risk factors after donation. These findings make us realize the importance of keeping long-term follow-up of donors to check for and prevent CKD risks even if their renal function remains stable for a long time, and to take immediate action if they develop these risks."

As I fumbled through the data, I expected to find at least one or two studies or reports that raised cause for concern. Because if donating an organ were so easy and risk-free, everyone would be doing it. Still, the study from Tokyo was not a red flag for me. Eight donors out of 1519 seemed like a margin of error, not the basis for me to walk away from the idea. Considering the odds of my being electrocuted were the same as the likelihood I would develop kidney disease later in life, I felt content with my research findings.[33] My intentions were still fully intact.

There was only one thing left for me to do: give the big pitch to my better half. Given that we didn't have any extreme medical conditions and were relatively young and nimble, we didn't think often about our mortality. For perfectly healthy people to volunteer for surgery wasn't something we were familiar with, but I felt Mat would understand my appeal and all the work I had done to arrive at my conclusion. Mat alone could make or break this idea, and he handled it just as I expected: he volleyed it back over to me.

I introduced the concept to him one night when he came home from work. Very matter-of-factly, I explained the Katie Couric episode about kidney chains, using my arms to flail around and simulate an airplane with a kidney onboard flying from one city to the next as the chain commenced. Then, I shared my corresponding research on the National Kidney Registry and the donors from across the country who had already done so.

Mat thought it was cool and sounded futuristic. He had never heard of such a concept either. When I told him that I wanted to see if I could give a kidney away, he didn't flinch. He just paused and looked at me and said, "Well, yeah, if you think this is a good idea, then you should check it out." He wondered why we had two kidneys if we didn't need them both, and what would happen if donors eventually needed a new kidney. I shared the studies showing how people with one kidney turn out just fine. Then I began a new list of questions to find answers to, beginning with "what if I need a kidney in the future? Do I get mine back?"

We've never been very conventional people, so his response to my big idea was also exactly as expected. We were the free spirits in our families from the moment we started dating, and we have supported each other in all things extreme and unusual. I think our destiny as a forever match was sealed after our house burned down in 1997. We were barely twenty when we were left houseless by faulty wiring behind an old kitchen cabinet. Due to insurance, we were able to stay at the local Holiday Inn Express until our new house was ready to move in. Seven months of living in those tight quarters forced us to grow closer than we might not have otherwise.

Our wedding in 2000 was next to a pond in the middle of a field, while the norm was to tend to those matters in a church, like proper Hoosiers. Going to college, global travels, and moving into leadership positions were all against the grain and contrary to what was expected of us. Still, we did it anyway because we supported each other in whatever wild and crazy ideas presented themselves. We've explored and conquered and climbed whatever mountain we chose to in our lives. And when your people lovingly refer to you as "the overachievers," it's not by accident. We own that, with pride.

I did not tell anyone but Mat about my interest in being a donor for a few reasons. Seeking personal opinions or asking permission to do as I pleased with my own body parts was never an essential factor in the choices I made. Also, at the time, I was a painfully private person. Talking about myself or my history was very difficult for me. In my profession, I was often in front of an audience, but I was discussing trade, jobs, and Congress, not my unconventional aspirations regarding the fate of my organs.

I felt like it might have sounded boastful if I were to tell friends I was thinking about doing this, and braggadocious I was not. Besides, I wasn't sure I wanted anyone to know about it to begin with. I can talk to you all day about surface-level stuff, but I'll stiffen right up if you want me to share my innermost thoughts. This was a personality trait I have carried my entire life, like a backpack chained to my shoulders with a lock and no key. My feelings and motivations have been buried deep down in the confines of my soul, never to surface. Exhibit A: It took me well over a decade to pull the words out of my internal archives to finish this book.

It was soon after my conversation with Mat that I got the ball rolling. I went to the National Kidney Registry website and clicked on the "I Want to Become a Kidney Donor" button. I submitted my name and contact information into the system and hit "send."

Naively, I presumed, since the need for kidneys was so dire, I'd have blood work completed to be sure a lifetime of Hamburger Helper didn't squash my chances at being a people helper and then be on an operating table in a matter of weeks. They'd rush me to the nearest hospital, and I'd bring new life to someone running out of hope just in time for the holidays. I would take it easy and ring in 2011 with one less organ in tow. No one would have to know, and my time off work would be muddled into the flurry of holiday vacation requests.

Sadly, this is not the timeline of how my story unfolded.

My impatience with all things that take entirely too long led me to believe that both of my kidneys were here to stay.

Chapter 6

# You Can't Hurry, Love

A few days after I submitted an inquiry on the National Kidney Registry website, I received a call from them, with an unidentified person on the other end. I'm sure they introduced themselves to me, but my mind, in a flurry of excitement, draws a blank now as to who they were and exactly what they said.

This is an unfortunate consequence of telling a tale years after it occurred. I don't have records, dates, or notes for some very meaningful aspects of this adventure, yet I retained pages of information about mundane segments of this process. For example, I have six copies of one set of bloodwork results but zero notes about the very first NKR person I spoke to on the phone that day.

The follow-up email I received to that unmemorable call instructed me to meet with my family doctor to order the initial tests I needed to qualify to become a donor. Attached to the email was a document titled *NKR Medical Certification Form*. It began, "I understand that I may be donating a kidney and as such, may be undergoing surgery…" It was just six sentences long and was, essentially, my contract acknowledging that I understood what I was attempting to do and that NKR would officially be my kidney's agent.

The physician section required my doctor, Dr. Kueber, to declare, as far as he knew, that I was of sound mind and body with no physical or mental issues that would prevent me from donating a kidney. Dr. Kueber and I both needed to sign it, then send it back to NKR with the results of the necessary labs that were listed at the bottom of the form.

Comprehensive Metabolic Panel

Urinalysis

24-hour Urine for Protein and Creatinine Clearance

Complete Blood Count

Hemoglobin A1C

Hepatitis Panel for A, AB, B, and C

To be of sound mind and body; that was an interesting declaration to note on the consent form. The reason I hadn't heard of people giving their kidneys away to people they didn't know before seeing it play out on Katie Couric's news segment was that it hadn't been a common occurrence. For starters, there wasn't a lot of interest within the medical community in bringing people like me and our kidneys into this equation for one simple reason: we must be psychotic.[34]

While no real data supported the notion that my insanity was leading me to give away my kidney, there was little to suggest I was sane either.[35] Non-directed donation was relatively new at the time, and there was sparse information to confirm or deny that I had all my faculties, despite wanting to donate an organ. Therein lies the rub.

My appointment was scheduled for November 29th, the soonest available. I was still hoping to accomplish my December donation goals, even as the 29th neared my own personal deadline for this process to begin. When I handed the paper to Dr. Kueber, he looked at it for what felt like an hour before he said, "You want to donate a kidney?"

Dr. Kueber had been our doctor for just a few years before this interaction, because our original doctor had retired and moved to Canada. We chose him because he had a holistic mind, suggesting food and vitamins over prescriptions in his treatment plans. He was close in age to us, and in addition to his practice, he worked at the local free clinic once a week. He was "good people" as far as we were concerned, and his question felt like less of a judgment than a piqued curiosity.

I explained to him about the Katie Couric episode, with my arms flailing around as I, again, simulated a kidney on board a plane as it flew to its new recipient. He looked intrigued, asked a few more questions, then left the room. I guessed he went to look NKR up on the internet to be sure I wasn't being looped into a black market for organ trafficking. When he came back, he smiled and commenced my physical. Eyes, ears, heart, reflexes, etc. He tapped on the keyboard and asked questions about my family that he had asked many times before. After proclaiming how interesting he thought the idea was, he signed the NKR form and handed me a paper to take to the lab.

The lab was located in one room inside Dr. Kueber's office and was the only lab in the small town of Garrett, Indiana. I gave my paperwork to the technician, who was always the only person I'd ever seen working there. She looked over the paper and commented that it was a big order. After I gave her a urine sample, she began filling endless vials with my blood. Then, she went into the closet, pulled out a big brown jug, and handed it to me. "This is for your 24-hour urine test," she said.

It was the same brown as a bottle of hydrogen peroxide. It was not quite the size of a gallon of milk, but not as small as a half-gallon either. The jug was somewhere in the middle of the two. My job was to put all my urine for 24 hours in that jug, and then bring it back to her.

That bottle was the most hysterical thing I'd seen in a while. Was that how much the average person pees in a day, nearly a gallon? I had no idea! And was I supposed to pee *into* it? The technician explained that the amount of urine people produce in a day varies, which is why the jug is so large. Some people can fill it up. I would need to use a standard urine sample cup and pour its contents into the jug. I would begin this test with the first urine of the morning and conclude it with the last urine of the night, before the next morning. I left the office, jug in hand, ready to get this party started.

The very next day, I began my 24-hour urine sample. I never imagined one person could pee enough to fill a jug of that size. Maybe Andre the Giant, but not me. Up until that point, I had never kept track of my pee-schedule. I just … peed. Surprisingly, however, when I returned the jug to the Lab Technician, it was nearly full. That must've meant my kidneys were uber-efficient at their jobs.

Two days later, my lab results were ready to be picked up from Dr. Kueber's office. So many pages. So many letters. So many numbers. It was all a jumbled mess of measurements I couldn't translate, other than my cholesterol numbers, which I prided myself on keeping low. Some tests were marked as "high" while others were "low", "abnormal", or "non-reactive." Perhaps having a "high" result on a kidney test meant I was overqualified and well above average. Or, as I suspected, all that Hamburger Helper and canned ravioli as a child showed up to haunt me on those pages.

I emailed the only address I had for NKR to see if I could scan the information over to them instead of using the mail. It was something generic like admin@kidneyregistry.org. A woman named Diane Zocchia emailed me back and wrote, "Yes, you can email them to me." Her signature line, which was in blue and italicized like mine, indicated she was the NKR Administrative Coordinator. She gave me her email address and fax number.

All my lab results and the signed medical certification form that Dr. Kueber and I signed were emailed to Diane on December 8th, 2010. Less than a month had passed since Katie Couric got the ball rolling for me, and there I was sealing the deal with my labs already in route. I was well on my way to a holiday hospital stay, I hoped.

The following week, Diane emailed to let me know my lab results would be sent to their medical board for review to see if I qualified to donate. She cautioned me that it sometimes takes a while to hear back from the board, but she would let me know as soon as she had news. Diane asked how far I was from Maywood, Illinois, because she hoped they could send me to Loyola University Medical Center for "my workup."

That email thoroughly deflated my December intentions. We were already in the second week of the month. I was not going to have this surgery before 2011 or ring in the new year with one kidney. And what are workups? I assumed the lab results I just sent in were proof of my stellar or not-so-stellar health. I was so naïve.

Maywood, Illinois, was about a four-hour drive from my house. Whatever a "workup" requires must be something fairly specific for NKR, not simply to have me go to my local lab or family doctor again. For me, four hours was a simple car ride. My job had conditioned me to sit in the driver's seat for long periods of time, so a short trip to Maywood was no big deal, and my brand-new UAW-made Ford Focus could get me anywhere. Just point the way!

On December 20th, Diane emailed to ask if I had time I could take off from work. Yes, I had vacation time and a few personal days that I could take when needed. If necessary, I could also have used sick leave or short-term disability, or called off for the day. I wasn't concerned with getting a day or two off to attend to this workup or a surgery. With my union advantage and my occupation, I had many options.

At that point in my career, I was working constantly to the extent that my work had become my life. For me, there was little distinction to be made between a day off and a day on the job, really. Given that I worked most of the time independently, I could rearrange my work assignments as necessary. I told Diane it was no sweat.

That December exchange with Diane was the last of my correspondence with NKR in 2010. Bread pudding, mashed potatoes, and beef and noodles consumed my attention for the remainder of the year, with my kidneys still existing within the same space. Since our old farmhouse was the largest in the family, many gatherings commenced there on an annual basis, and that year was no exception. Mat and I hosted three holiday dinners that month, then took nearly a dozen of our nieces and nephews on an adventure across Northern Indiana. No one was the wiser about my kidney crusade.

On January 5, 2011, Diane requested additional tests. The medical board wanted the urinalysis, urine culture, 24-hour urine collection, creatinine clearance, and hepatitis C antibody tests repeated. She wasn't told why the tests needed to be repeated, but she said it wasn't an unusual request. A lot of times, when tests are repeated, the results are better, she explained.

A trip to the hospital lab was in order this time, as it was conveniently located near my house. There, I received yet another jug to piss in. It again made me chuckle to walk out to my car with that giant bottle. I wondered if I had done something wrong with the first jug, which required me to repeat the test. How many ways are there to pee in a jug, really? By the end of February, I had a new set of lab results sent to Diane. They once again had all the necessary dirt on my innards.

In March, I received the summary of benefits from my insurance company for all of the lab work I had. I was fortunate to have what, at the time of the Affordable Care Act debate, was nicknamed a "Cadillac plan." Benefits like mine were cherished. Folks held onto their jobs for dear life, as dreadful as some of them may have been, to carry the same golden ticket I had. I knew I was one of the lucky ones. Over $800 in lab work didn't cost me anything out of pocket. It was completely covered. The re-checks cost $63. I wondered how the "workup at Loyola" lurking in the future would be paid for. I could handle a $63 bill here and there, but had no idea what expenses I was in for. That was another question for my new list: "What's this workup going to cost me?"

How would people with limited means or mediocre insurance manage to do any of this? How many people looked at their lab bills and decided against going any further in the donation process because they couldn't afford to help? Nearly a decade would pass before I learned of the national movement to compensate living donors, which I wholeheartedly supported.

Spring came. Spring went. I continued to go through the motions of my life as the status of my kidneys remained unknown. I taught trade workshops for the Steelworkers Union at the University of Illinois. Congress got a visit from yours truly on the importance of the multiplier effect of manufacturing jobs in their districts. I worked with interfaith groups in South Bend, Indiana; Unitarian Universalists in Midland, Michigan; and Manufacturing Extension Partnerships in Orlando, Florida. We celebrated Mat's graduation from college, and his trip to volunteer as tech support in Haiti after the 7.0 earthquake came and went. Life continued to happen. By design, my life was so busy that I forgot I was even waiting on anything. On July 22, the news finally came.

Hi Rachel,

We finally heard back from our medical board.

They have approved you to move on to the next step, which would be to coordinate your workup at one of our participating transplant centers. Kindly go to our website to the Transplant

Centers tab. There you will find a list of all of our participating transplant centers. Please review it and let me know which center would be the most convenient for you to go to.

Once you let me know, I will get in touch with them to schedule your workup.

If you have any questions, please don't hesitate to contact me.

Have a nice weekend!

Diane

Moving on to the next step sounded exciting. Still, I was curious to know just how many steps were involved in this process, since eight months had already passed since I clicked the button on the NKR website. Is this why so many people die waiting? Is this why so many people don't donate?

Side note: The Evolution of Kidney Donation

*In 2010, the National Kidney Registry and non-directed kidney donation as a whole were like a fresh coat of paint: they needed time to show their shine. Best practices and processes, as well as participating transplant hospitals, were all evolving as the concept of chain reactions with organs gained traction. My uber-impatience in those early years was real. But little did I know or appreciate that all of these professionals were simply trying to make the best decisions for everyone involved. Donating a kidney is now a much more streamlined process.*

# Chapter 7

# **What If...**

The weekend I received Diane's email, I was in Granite City, Illinois. My pal Ed Sadlowski received the Steelworker SOAR Lifetime Achievement Award, and I went to celebrate and to work. From the comfort of my hotel room, I perused the NKR website to pick a hospital. The webpage contained listings from across the country, including statistics on the number of transplants each had performed through the chain program. Choosing which hospital to do my workup could, by default, result in having my surgery at that same hospital, if we ever arrived at that intersection.

For the Midwest, there were limited options nearby. At the time, not a single hospital in Indiana was listed on the NKR site. The closest were in Cleveland, Ohio, and Maywood, Illinois. My sister and her family still lived near Cleveland in our hometown, and I had several family members and friends in and around that region. It would be nice to have them close if I were to have surgery. I didn't know anyone in Maywood, but I had a few pals in the Chicagoland region, including Ed.

Looking at the number of transplants each hospital performed with NKR, Loyola University Medical Center in Maywood surpassed the Cleveland option by a wide margin. In my mind, that meant they did more transplant surgeries overall, so they were obviously the best choice. Being in unchartered territory, I had to consider more than just the hospital's location. My perception of their "seniority in the factory" played a factor as well.

When I got home after the weekend and talked it over with Mat, we decided to go with Loyola. It seemed like the best choice, and

Diane mentioned it months ago in her emails to me. I let her know of my choice, and also that I already had a few upcoming work commitments that I could not reschedule. Diane explained that the coordinators at Loyola would call me to schedule my workup, which would take three or four days to complete. NKR would assist with any travel and lodging arrangements I needed.

This "workup" process must be really something. My mind wandered through the universe of possibilities to understand what kinds of things I would be doing to require multiple days in a hospital setting. Maybe I'd have to run an obstacle course to check my endurance, or perhaps I'd need to sleep in some sort of hyperbaric chamber to test my functions. An aptitude test? Or would I need to document the history of what my kidneys have been through? I didn't ask Diane what a workup was. I was excited about the unknown, but still wondering how many more unknowns there'd be and if my kidney would ever fly the coop.

Weeks passed before Barb Thomas called me from Loyola. She was friendly and happy to hear that I would be coming to Loyola for my testing. Once I explained my scheduling conflicts, we settled on October 16-19, nearly three months into the future. This was the only pocket of time they had available for my workup that didn't conflict with my work trips. Finally, a date had been set.

In late August, I received an "informed consent" document in the mail to sign, along with my schedule for the upcoming October trip. The schedule was signed by Joanna Czemske, listed as the "Donor Kidney Transplant Coordinator." I bet that was a pretty rewarding occupation. Typically, bad things bring people to the hospital: death, strokes, broken bones. Birthing babies and organ transplants are the few rays of sunlight that exist in a place like that.

Also included in my packet were instructions for yet another 24-hour urine sample. The four-day work-up would begin with me filling the jug on Sunday and bringing it with me to the hospital lab. Six different appointments would commence over the course of four days: a skin test, an EKG, an angiogram, a psychiatric evaluation with a psychiatrist, and a meeting with a doctor. My last appointment before leaving the hospital would be with the surgeon and patient advocate.

A psychiatrist. I had spent my life purposefully hoarding my thoughts and feelings. A mandatory visit to a psychiatrist was not something I was looking forward to. Grana was the only person to regularly talk about the hard stuff, and the Sicilian blood running through my veins, thanks to Dad's side of the gene pool, ensured my capacity to lock my thoughts and feelings away was strong. I had hoped that the meeting would be a simple check of my faculties: to ask me what year it was and if I knew where my kidneys were located, rather than inquiring about how I felt about the world and my place within it. Keeping it strictly to kidney talk would be very much appreciated. All other aspects of my life and experiences were not on the table.

I wondered if "the surgeon" would be the person who would eventually perform the surgery. Perhaps their name wasn't included in the list because they hadn't chosen that person yet, or maybe it was left out intentionally for confidentiality reasons. There weren't names listed for anyone on the appointment sheet, except Dr. Vavra for my primary care appointment and one other: "Tell the clerk you need lab work, an EKG, and a chest x-ray for Dr. Milner."

I imagined the patient advocate to be like a union steward. At my factory, I had served as a shop steward for many years. It's a thankless job to tussle with the bosses on behalf of your coworkers, ensuring that management treats everyone fairly. You could develop a reputation that you either need to uphold or defend. On the one hand, your coworkers never feel like you're doing enough to protect them; at the same time, you are the only one standing in the way of the boss running them over with a forklift, figuratively speaking, of course.

To advocate for a patient, just as one would advocate for a worker on the shop floor, was something I could fully appreciate. However, I was curious exactly why one would need a patient advocate in a transplant situation. I mean, we're all playing on the same team here, aren't we? However, having this position embedded in a donor program was quite honorable and intrigued me.

I worked with Diane on the logistics of my trip. She booked the LaQuinta Inn in Oakbrook Terrace, near the hospital. I would be working nearby, speaking at the racial equality and economic justice conference held by the A. Philip Randolph Institute, which meant I only had a one-hour drive to get there. NKR would reimburse me for the gas and tolls incurred during my commute. They would also reimburse me for meals. My responsibility was to simply get there, with my jug-full of urine. NKR would take care of the rest.

Since it felt like this process and my involvement in it were getting down to the nitty-gritty, we finally decided to tell the parents and my sister. I hated talking about myself. Even sharing this news made me cringe. It was all about me. No amount of deflecting could be done to talk about my kidney without all roads leading to the owner of it.

For the parents, we did this casually, almost in passing, the next time we saw them. My plan was not to cause too much of a scene or excitement with the news. I didn't want any of them to go into panic mode. At that point, I felt they should be given a heads-up on what I was thinking about doing, you know, as an FYI.

I said something like, "I'm looking into donating a kidney through this program that does chain reactions. It sounds cool. Can you pick up some dog food for me when you go into town? Thanks...."

Mat's mom, Deb, asked good questions, and I navigated through the conversation well with her. She thought it was an awesome thing to do. She was, by nature, a good person to break any news to. Affectionately dubbed "the town listener," she could handle much of anything people unleashed on her, and she did so with a smile. If I told her I was joining the circus or running for President, she'd offer up the same encouraging words.

Mat's dad and stepmom, Mike and Ruth, took their time to process what I was saying. You could see the gears shifting and the emergence of anxiety on their faces. Still, they just nodded their heads. By then, they had grown accustomed to hearing unconventional ideas and adventurous tales from us. Still, everyone has an opinion, and at that point, they kept theirs, whatever it may have been, all to themselves.

Dad handled the news exactly as I suspected he would: he played defense. The questions he asked were accusatory, as if I were ten and had just spilled the milk: "Why do you want to do that?" "What if the one you keep goes bad?" "What if someone in the family needs one later? Then what?" Dad's wife, Kay, had a few good questions but remained neutral on the matter. That was her very diplomatic way of keeping the peace.

When I told Grana, she asked if I would have to take pills after surgery. When I explained that nothing would change for me after my donation, she nodded her head and said, "Okay." This was not news to be worked up over, in her eyes. She knew from decades past how important organ donation was, starting with the death of my Uncle Ed. Grana had complete confidence in me to make the right choices for my own body parts.

Just as I wanted to toss the idea out there and quickly change the subject, so did my sister. After I gave Dara the two-second pitch on the phone, she then told me about her trip to the Salvation Army on half-off Wednesday. And that was that. Being raised by a single dad for much of our lives, who was himself raised in a family of Italian Americans of Sicilian persuasion, enabled Dara and me to inherit the prime thing this demographic does very well; they don't talk about things.

Dad played defense because he had been the lone protector and the parent. He and the grandmas and the aunts in our family had gotten us all the way into adulthood relatively unscathed. And there I was telling him I planned to throw a wrench in it. I was going to put my life at risk for someone I didn't know, a life he'd worked so hard to protect.

I didn't blame him for having that reaction. I understood it and expected it from him. If I had a kid tell me something like that, I might have had the same feelings on the inside. You want to protect your kids from harm, even when they are fully grown adults. And when you think they are intentionally placing themselves in it, well, I guess it can make you go bananas.

My pal Mike was in on the scoop early in this adventure. He became my most cherished friend in our work lives. He and I worked together most frequently among our coworkers, traveling far and wide to promote manufacturing. As a retired local union president, Mike was a skilled conversationalist and listener. He had nothing but interest and kindness to give me about my kidney crusade. He was also the person I'd be working with in Gary before heading to Loyola to do my work-up. He would know something was awry even if I didn't tell him.

A week before my Loyola appointments, I received a letter from Joanna in the mail. Enclosed was a one-page flyer about UNOS, along with a document I had to sign and mail back to her to acknowledge receipt. *OPTN/UNOS: Your Resource for Organ Transplant Information.* It included a toll-free number I could call with questions about donations. It seemed like a helpline or customer service program to ensure that any concerns I had could be addressed.

On Sunday, the official start of my work-up, I lounged in the La Quinta Inn, filling the jug and preparing for my appointments. I had accumulated about a dozen questions to be answered by one or all the people I'd be meeting during the visits. I had them jotted down and ready to ask. Some of the questions I had researched and already knew the answers to, but in all things, it's best to verify.

To give myself extra inspiration, I explored a few articles I found about Loyola's kidney program. By all accounts, it was an impressive outfit, a leader in the field. In March 2010, the first-ever kidney chain in Illinois took place at Loyola, with three people stepping forward to donate kidneys to strangers since the program's inception.[36] In June 2010, the first-ever living donor kidney to be flown into Chicago was received by Lilian Rosa, a Loyola patient who was part of a chain. That chain continued with her husband, Jose, paying it forward by donating his kidney to a stranger. By June, Loyola had 21 non-directed donors enrolled in its program.[37]

In April 2011, Loyola made headlines with yet another milestone in kidney donation. Seven Loyola staff members, dubbed the "Seven Sisters," became kidney donors, enabling 28 people to receive transplants.[38] To have that many donors in one workplace had been unprecedented until the women emerged. One of them was Barb Thomas, the same person who scheduled my work-up appointments.

One of the "Sisters," Dorothy Jambrosek, summed up their intent so perfectly in the article. "We are ordinary people," said Jambrosek.

"But because of us, twenty-eight dialysis-dependent people's lives have been changed. We hope that [our example] is a call to action. We believe there are others like us who can make a difference." Dorothy saw herself in the same light as I did. "We are ordinary people" working toward something extraordinary, a movement of compassion. Every article I read mentioned Dr. John Milner, head of this, director of that, founder of all things kidney in Chicago. For sure, I was destined to meet this guy, maybe as soon as Monday.

Bright and early on Monday, October 17, 2011, I arrived at the Loyola campus. It was 6:30 am, and I was running on empty. They had instructed me not to eat or drink anything for twelve hours prior. I always feel grumpy when my morning schedule is detoured. Waking up with coffee and the news always helped me start the day off right. But on October 17, I had to make an exception.

I arrived bearing a priceless gift. With the giant 24-hour urine jug in my bag, someone was sure to be pleased to receive it. As my third completed jug in this process, I hoped it would be my last. My first appointment in the lab was where I delivered the jug, and finally said goodbye to yesterday's pee.

My workup began with extensive lab work. They took vial after vial from my arm. And more urine. I had an EKG and a chest x-ray, then I was on my way to the third floor for a skin test. It was a PPD (purified protein derivative) test that determined whether someone had tuberculosis. I then went back downstairs to radiology to have a 3D CT angiogram. So many words. So many tests.

I had never had an angiogram, but it felt very much like an MRI. I lay on a table that slid into the middle of a giant machine with a hole in the center, like a big donut hole. The very frazzled but personable radiologist had a terrible time finding a good vein for me. Because the needle used to inject the dye was so large, the vein she used had to be large as well. If the vein was too small, she explained, the pressure from the dye going in could cause it to rupture.

Of all the times I gave blood, I never had a problem with finding a good vein. But this needle she was trying to use was gargantuan, like a crochet needle, a BBQ skewer, a Phillips screwdriver. Finally, a vein cooperated, and I was swiftly conveyed into the donut hole. I could feel the dye as it began to flow through my body. It was hot. I lay there as still as I could, hoping that feeling was normal and trying to prevent a vein "blow-out" from occurring. Just like an MRI, it sounded like the machine was breaking as it squeaked and churned out its results. Then, I was done.

Considering my poor sense of direction and accumulated anxiety about sharing my feelings, I was under considerable stress trying to locate my next appointment. The Department of Psychiatry was in a building on the other side of the hospital campus. It was so far away that a shuttle was advised.

The appointment sheet noted that I had to arrive 30 minutes early and that if I did not, they would not see me. Further, it noted they might not reschedule another appointment for me if I were late. What this conveyed to me, as an apprehensive, mandatory patient, was that the Department of Psychiatry, in its entirety, was an asshole. The tone and my opposition to talking about myself had me going into this appointment entirely offended by a building, a department, and a psychiatrist I had never met.

I took a deep breath and sat down. There was no leather couch to be laid upon, just three chairs, two of which were occupied. I don't recall what either of the women looked like or their names. Both were taking notes. They were there to evaluate me to determine if I was of sound mind to give away an organ. For my part, I tried to remain positive that I'd make it out of that room, being declared a fully functioning person who knew what date it was and that my kidneys were on either side of my spine, right below my ribcage.

They began asking me basic questions about myself, such as my occupation, education, and health. They asked how I came to the decision to donate a kidney and if I understood the donation process. I told them about the questions I had to ask the surgeon at my appointment and that I was looking forward to becoming a donor.

Once they switched gears to ask about my family history, my heart sank into my gut. I sensed, by the end of the day, my "kidney application" would have a big red stamp on it: DENIED.

"Tell me about your father's health."

"He's fine."

"And your mother?"

"She's dead."

"How did she die?"

It's the slant of the head, the pursing of the lips, the familiar look of pity on the faces of those who learn of my mother's death that enrages me. I've lived my entire life seeing this type of face staring back at me. When Dara and I were out in public with Grana, she'd always introduce us as "Joy's daughters," leaving the person on the other end of that exchange to instantly react with remorse, as if we were the ones who died. Parent-teacher conferences in school and holiday events with extended family always led to people connecting us to death, except we were very much alive, for crying out loud. They say that anger in women often manifests in the form of tears. I know this as fact. I know this very well.

I don't talk about my mother on purpose. And when I'm forced to, I feel as if I now bear the burden and the responsibility of her battles, of her identity, of her consequences. This is why my feelings stay tucked into the confines of my soul, only to surface when I'm forced to spill my guts in a mandatory psych review. By the time I left that meeting, I was exhausted and defeated. My plan to be a donor had surely caught a snag. I was thoroughly pissed that my health could very well be stellar, but my family tree may stop me in my tracks.

Doesn't everyone have baggage, though? Show me someone without some traumatic family event or closeted skeleton, and I'll show you a liar. Trauma and pain are not exclusive to my gene pool. It's quite possible to come from a fragmented home and still want to help save the world in some small way. If every potential donor like me were ruled out because of our baggage, more people would die. I hoped those women, with their pens, notepads, and pity-filled faces, understood that.

I spent the next day lounging around my hotel room, reflecting on the intermittent road I'd traveled to get that far in the donor workup.

The schedulers purposely left Tuesday open so that if I missed any appointments on Monday, I would have the following day to make them up. With one day left to meet with a doctor, surgeon, and patient advocate, I still had a chance to advance to the next round of this process.

Doctor Vavra was a family doctor. His role in this process was to ask all the same questions my doctor back home, Dr. Kueber, would ask. He took the hammer to my knees, looked in my ears, felt around my neck, and listened to me breathe. He checked my skin where they did the TB test on Monday. If the bubble under the skin spread beyond a specific diameter, it indicated a person had Tuberculosis. My bubble got bigger, but was neither outside of the lines nor inside. It was somewhere in the middle. He ordered another blood test for me just to be sure.

On the third floor of the urology department, I met people who were intimately connected to this process. Joanna Czemske, donor kidney transplant coordinator, greeted me as I arrived. Barb Thomas, the scheduler, a kidney donor herself, was also there.

I met other people who held various titles: Roseann Ghusein was a social worker and donor coordinator, like Joanna. Janice Papp, also a social worker, was my designated patient advocate. This was all clear as mud. An organizational family tree diagram would have been extremely helpful to me during this first meeting. There were so many people holding so many different, but intermingling roles. I couldn't keep them all straight, but finally, I could put faces to names.

With my notebook in hand, I headed into an empty exam room and waited. Soon, a white-coated man walked in and extended his hand to shake mine.

"Hi Rachel, I'm John Milner. Thanks for coming all this way."

The infamous Dr. Milner and I were finally in the same room. After reading all those articles featuring him, he almost seemed like a celebrity. He looked close to my age and had an energy about him, as if he was high on life. I suppose, with a job like his, how could you not be?

Dr. Milner had a very personable way of speaking. We had more of a conversation than a wonky review of kidney surgery. One of the first things he remarked on was my cholesterol numbers, which had always been Oscar-worthy. I explained how my family collectively tracked our numbers for years to keep tabs and also bully each other to be healthy. That might have been a first for him. As I went through my questions, he answered every one of them with as much information as I could digest. He talked. I took notes.

### *What if I need a kidney later in life? Do I get mine back?*

As a living donor, I would be moved to the top of the kidney transplant waitlist, right below kids, should I ever need one in the future. My own kidney, which would have been living and working in another person's body, would not be given back to me. It didn't work that way.

There was a 1 in 1,500 chance that a donor would ever need a kidney in their lifetime, and not due to donation. That was the rate at which the average population needed a kidney. Because kidney donors are healthy enough to give away a kidney, they are healthier than the average person to begin with. If the tests revealed I was far from average, this statistic wouldn't apply.

Most people in their lifetime never get the workup that potential kidney donors receive. Transplant centers need to ensure we are fully able to function with one kidney and give away another pristine kidney as well, which is why more than $30,000 in tests would be done to make sure of that.

### *How much of this process will I have to pay for?*

None of the expenses for surgery or the pre-testing would be my responsibility. Once a recipient is identified, all costs will be covered by that person's insurance. Because I had signed up with NKR, receipts for food, gas, and hotels should be sent to them for reimbursement. Dr.

Milner also mentioned an insurance policy that NKR offered, which he said I should ask about.

### *What are the complications after surgery?*

A blood pressure increase of about five points can occur in donors later in life. However, modifying the diet can help control it. There is a 3 in 10,000 death rate among donors after surgery. This was primarily due to the use of a "wet clip," which caused internal bleeding. At Loyola, the wet clips were not used. There was a 1 in 1,000 chance of getting blood clots in my legs after surgery due to immobility.

### *What percent of kidneys are rejected?*

There was a 1% chance that a kidney would be rejected by its recipient.

### *When can I return to work?*

After I told Dr. Milner what kind of work I did, he said I should be able to return to work 10 to 12 days after surgery. Because I lived so far away from Loyola, they'd require me to stay nearby at a motel for a week after surgery, in case of any complications. If I needed pain medication, I couldn't drive while I was using it, of course. Any lifting over ten pounds would need to wait for a few months.

### *What are the transplant statistics for Loyola?*

The average wait time to find a match in the NKR system was 2 months, compared to years of waiting on the national list. The previous year, Loyola had 11 chains, beginning with a donor like me, resulting in 70 transplants nationwide. Five of those 11 donors were staff members, from the "Seven Sisters." Of those eleven chains, nine also ended at Loyola, with the last donor in a chain giving to the last recipient at their center. If Loyola starts a chain by giving away the first kidney, it typically receives the last one in the chain as reciprocation for initiating the chain.

Nine patients who were children or had a high probability of rejection were also transplanted as part of the program, which gave hope to those who had completely lost all hope. Since 2008, just three years earlier, NKR had facilitated nearly 400 transplants, with 68 non-directed donors from across the country.

### *How are surgeries timed?*

The whole program is at the mercy of the donor. They offer donors like me the choice to set the surgery date, and every other process and corresponding surgery will work around that date. Because none of it would be possible without that one person, the donor calls the shots.

The donor can set the surgery date, but they also have the option to cancel it. Until the time a person is rolled into surgery, they can still change their mind. A donor can decide to keep their kidney and go home fully intact, leaving every other potential donor and recipient also to have their surgeries cancelled.

### *What about coffee? I need my coffee.*

I can eat and drink anything I want, all in moderation.

Dr. Milner then turned the tables. He had questions for me that he needed to ask to help me think about different scenarios in case any of them ever happened. I didn't need to answer them immediately or even know that they might occur, but these catastrophic events and my feelings about them had to be taken into consideration.

What if you donate your kidney and you never hear from the recipient? How would you feel?

What if your kidney is on its way to its recipient and the plane crashes? You've just lost your kidney, and no one else benefits from your loss. How would you feel?

What if your kidney gets lost in transit? How would you feel?

What if your kidney fails and the recipient needs another one? How would you feel?

What if your future child or a loved one needs a kidney?

What if you need a kidney in the future? How would you feel about your donation?

Dr. Milner's questions gave me some very critical things to consider. How *would* I feel if I never learned whether my kidney was serving someone well? Did I feel a certain obligation to hear from the recipient since I gave them my organ? Maybe I did. I mean, shouldn't a simple thank-you card be expected out of this exchange? He explained that a gift as significant as a kidney is not something that everyone can put into words, and when it comes from a perfect stranger who steps up to give it, the difficulty is magnified. I would have to accept that if I never heard from the recipient, they just couldn't find the words.

I must admit, some of these transportation twists I hadn't imagined happening. How does a kidney "get lost"? Who does Loyola work with: a carrier pigeon? And, sure, a plane could crash, but the odds of that happening are in the zillions. I'd be equally distraught about all the passengers who also crashed as I would be about my kidney on board.

Since Mat and I committed to not having children, we weren't concerned with "saving ours" for them. But we did have a couple of dozen kids in our lives that were equally important. If any of them needed a kidney, I would expect another family member or someone like me to step forward to help them, just as I was doing. Holding onto a kidney just in case a family member needed one was illogical to me, considering that need may never come. Doing so would mean I missed an opportunity to help someone when they really needed me, all for nothing, for a "what if."

The power to change your mind up until you enter the surgical ward was comforting, but at the same time, horrifying. To build up the hope and excitement of so many people, only to be so scared that you change your mind, was hard for me to imagine. Was there a mechanism in the brain that causes this to happen to everyday folks like me? Could I be the person who gets cold feet and lets people down? Damn, I sure hope not.

I knew I only had control over certain things in order to maintain my own personal health. Diet, exercise, and lifestyle could help me live my healthiest life, but not everything was within my control. I could only do so much to stay healthy, with one or two kidneys. The rest depended on the stars aligning, Mother Nature sprinkling me with magic dust, or the unknown writers of the script we call life, including it in the storyline.

Given the damage Randy "Macho Man" Savage had done to his kidneys every time he got pummeled in the ring, my best bet to ensure I didn't lose my remaining kidney would be to avoid becoming a professional wrestler. There would be no kidney punches in the ring for me. Nope, no pissing blood on my watch. I planned to continue living my life fully present and to refrain from joining the World Wrestling Federation.

Chapter 8

# It Was Officially Official

The 100-page booklet I took home, "Partnering with Your Transplant Team: A Patient's Guide to Transplantation," looked vintage.[39] It was a 2008 publication by the U.S. Department of Health, geared toward the experiences of individuals in need of a transplant. Inside were sections for writing notes, jotting down important contacts, and recording lab results. It also had a section about deceased donation, which is how most organ recipients would receive their gifts of life. There was an organizational chart detailing all the involved organ donation agencies in the country. A list of costs a recipient should consider was also included.

"Few patients are able to pay all transplant costs from a single source. For example, you may be able to finance the transplant procedure through insurance coverage and pay for other expenses through savings accounts or by selling your assets."

There was a very brief mention of living donation in two sections of the booklet. A total of eight sentences explained this as an option if blood relatives were eligible to donate. Unrelated donors could also donate "if the transplant hospital approves." On the first page of the Appendix, at the very back, on page 83, a short fact was listed.

"Did you know? In 2007, more than 2,400 living organ donations were made between unrelated (non-biological) donors and recipients. Kidney donation is the most common living organ donation."

I was also given a brochure titled "Living Donation: Information You Need to Know.[40]" It contained everything that would have been oh so useful to learn before my appointment. While it was only a twelve-page booklet, it provided a comprehensive overview of what I was getting into, including the specifics of what a "workup" entailed, recovery from the surgery, and financial and insurance considerations. The Dr. Seuss quotation on the last page of the brochure really struck me.

"To the world you may be one person, but to one person you may be the world."

It turns out that donating a kidney could be a negative attribute in the eyes of the life and health insurance industries. My missing kidney might be considered a pre-existing condition, prompting an increase in my premiums. While this brochure was printed during the heated uncertainty over the Affordable Care Act, President Obama had already, by this time, protected me on the health insurance front. For life insurance, I wasn't so sure.

Grana bought life insurance policies for all four of us grandkids when we were very young. She was a protector and a planner, let me tell you. We each received whole life insurance policies with a $50,000 face value that cost an easy $120 a year to maintain. I couldn't imagine needing any more insurance than what I already had from her. At least, they couldn't take that away.

As I reviewed Dr. Milner's questions from my appointment, one of them stuck in my mind like a familiar song. One that I needed to pay special attention to. "What if your future child or a loved one needs a kidney, then what?" I inventoried the files in my brain to be sure I wasn't missing anything or anyone. Then, a key memory resurfaced that I had completely forgotten; Dad might need my kidney.

Years ago, I was conducting a local union training in Lima, Ohio, with my coworker, Randy. That experience was traumatic for both of us, initially for very different reasons. It was one of the first trainings I co-led for my union, which required a lot of preparation and planning on my part. During our week there, Randy had suffered a heart attack. With 100% blockage of his artery, the widow maker almost took his life. I had never been a bystander to a heart attack happening before my eyes. We had to act fast and stay calm.

Lucky for us, my lead foot and superior driving abilities, Randy's sense of direction, and the local hospital saved his life. Out of that experience came the revelation that tests exist to detect calcification long before a heart attack could strike. The Electron Beam Computed Tomography (EBCT) test provides a glimpse of any abnormalities in the general heart region. And for the low, low price of $99, anyone could get one.

For Christmas later that year, like a couple of weirdos, Mat and I bought ourselves and each of our parents that test. As peculiar as it sounds, as a family, we went to Parkview Memorial Hospital, and one by one, we were pushed into an MRI-like machine to have a look under the hood. We all came out of that experience with a typical diagnosis: we were all fine, except Dad. A few days after our Christmas field trip, someone from Parkview called him. They said his heart looked fine, but they saw a growth on his kidney. Dad made an appointment with his family doctor, who checked him over and declared that cysts come and go, and he had nothing to worry about.

This happened many years ago, and Dad's doctor said he was fine. Still, I wanted to be doubly sure. Had it not been for Dr. Milner's question about my own kidney, I would have forgotten all about that trip to the hospital and Dad's test results. I asked Dad to go back to his doctor and make sure his kidneys were okay. My kidney was going to be donated either way, provided I passed my own tests, but Dad would get first dibs if he needed it. His recheck with the doctor went well. Dad wouldn't need my kidney after all, but he was not interested in hearing about me giving it away either.

A few weeks after my workup appointments, I sent Diane a spreadsheet and copies of my receipts for the time I was in Maywood. She said NKR would reimburse me for everything, even that late-night smoothie. My three-day trip totaled $115.12, excluding the hotel, which Diane had already arranged and paid for.

Janice Papp, a Loyola social worker and patient advocate, began paperwork to see if I qualified for financial assistance through the National Living Donor Assistance Center (NLDAC). They helped people afford to donate by assisting with travel and meals for follow-up and clinic visits related to donation. It's an income-based program, so not everyone is eligible to receive help paying for expenses, and various conditions must be met.

NKR was paying for my expenses regardless of my ability to pay for them myself, which was a welcome incentive for me or anyone considering donation. I wondered if people outside of the NKR program could afford to pay these costs and just how rigid those NLDAC conditions were. Sure, financially well-off donors would be just fine taking on those expenses, but was the donor pool full of them, or was it full of donors like me teetering somewhere in the middle?

In November, at Dr. Milner's request, Joanna asked me to conduct additional tests. I needed an ultrasound of my thyroid because Dr. Vavra thought he felt an enlarged thyroid gland during my October exam. An appointment with an infectious disease doctor was also needed because my skin test for tuberculosis was on the margins. Once again, I needed to meet with a psychiatrist because the one I met with in October felt I was not fully informed about what I was signing up for.

Another dreaded psych visit: just what I was hoping not to have to repeat. Joanna had been reaching out to a hospital closer to me to arrange the visits, so I wouldn't have to drive to Maywood again, but they were unresponsive to her repeated calls and emails. I offered to reach out to them myself if it would help expedite the process. By December, Diane finally asked me to return to Loyola to undergo the additional tests. NKR would again pay my expenses.

On January 4th, 2012, I was scheduled for my second trip to Loyola. My appointment sheet came in the mail. I had enough time to drive from home on the morning of the 4th, attend to the follow-up appointments, and make it home that evening. There would be no overnights or big jugs to piss in this time. Two medical exams and one psychiatrist, presumably shining a laser beam into my soul, trying to find my inner demons, were on the agenda.

I spent yet another November birthday with both of my kidneys. It was meant to be my 2010 gift to the world, but there I was at the end of 2011, still fully intact. That makes two birthday gifts that this one kidney now has to fulfill. Perhaps I can consider the amount of hustle and research it took in 2010 as my gift for that year, and the number of urine jugs I gave to the medical industry as my golden gift for 2011.

Will my actual kidney be the 2012 gift? Stay tuned for News at 11.

That December, we took Mat's dad, Ruth, my dad, and Kay out for a holiday dinner. At a local fundraiser, we had won dinner for six in the President's quarters of the university where Mat worked. As we were treated to a four-course meal, complete with multiple fork choices, medallions of butter, and tiny sugar cubes, I gave them an update on my kidney.

Silence.

Aside from Kay asking about the specifics of my upcoming appointment in January, no one had anything to say. Perhaps they were all still hoping I'd change my mind or that one of these appointments would somehow rule me out. Then, they could breathe a collective sigh of relief. We changed the subject for the rest of the meal, and that was fine by me.

My January 4th appointments at Loyola went as I expected. The ultrasound of my thyroid showed nothing alarming. The infectious disease doctor asked a lot of questions about my travels across the globe to Australia, Japan, China, and Brazil. Knowing my destinations helped him gauge whether I could have picked up something sketchy that caused my TB test to be inconclusive. He, too, cleared me of any concern.

I stayed as frozen as a snowwoman in the psychiatry office. The doctor asked me about the donation process. She asked me if I understood what I was signing up for. She could read how annoyed I was to be in that room again, I'm sure. I was an uncooperative patient. There was no spilling of my guts to be done, as patients who visited this office on purpose might want to do. Nope, not today.

My receipts for the January 4th trip were again sent to Diane for reimbursement by NKR. They totaled $90.31, primarily for tolls.

In mid-February, Roseann Ghusein, whom I'd first met in October, called me. I had finally been approved to be a donor. I was excited about the news, but I was still unsure how long the road ahead would be. If it took as long to find a match as it did to clear me to donate, my kidney could shrivel up by then. Roseann would keep me posted on my status once they entered my data into the NKR matching system.

Shortly after our call, I received a letter from Loyola, which made it official. It was signed by Roseann on behalf of Dr. Milner.

*Dear Rachel,*

*The gift you want to give is truly a very precious and selfless act. Thank you for your patience during our thorough evaluation process. It is our duty to be sure that your health is not compromised and that you are protected from potential harm. Your case was presented to the Donor Selection Committee for discussion and evaluation on February 7, 2012.*

*We are pleased to inform you that you have been approved as a living kidney donor. As previously discussed, you will be entered into the NKR system, and we will keep you posted.*

Being medically cleared to donate was a huge step in this process. It made things seem very real. Up until that February call, I was looking to donate a kidney. I wanted to donate a kidney. I was trying to donate a kidney. But just like that, I was officially qualified to do so. There's no wiggle room from that. I couldn't wake up one day and say I changed my mind about exploring the option. No, the option had been explored to death. It was explored, then explored some more. It was explored to its successful conclusion. I was medically cleared: no takebacks.

I felt a bit anxious for a minute. This was really going to happen. All that Hamburger Helper and factory pollution wasn't enough to disqualify me. No amount of Lake Erie contaminants or family baggage was going to rain on my donation parade. I must have been invincible all along and didn't even know it. This thing I had been working toward and thinking about for fifteen months had reached a monumental peak.

A week later, I received a package in the mail from Loyola. It contained empty tubes that needed to be filled with my blood. I was to go to my local lab, have my blood drawn, and then send the tubes to the HLA lab at Loyola for testing. HLA type testing (Human Leukocyte Antigen) is what determines your "type" in order to identify who else in the world is also your "type.[41]" Much like a marriage matchmaking service, but for kidneys.

I went to the lab in Dr. Kueber's office, where most of my lab tests had been conducted for years as a patient. The tech looked over my sheet from Loyola. At the top, it read "Kidney Donor" and instructed her to send them the bill instead of charging me. She looked at the handful of tubes that needed to be filled and said, "If you're going to donate a kidney, the least I can do is draw your blood. I won't bother with a bill."

It wasn't long after sending my blood through the mail that Roseann called me with news. A match was identified. If I were looking at Roseann when she gave me that news, I bet her face would be void of muscle activation. Her tone was completely neutral, as if she were calling to renew my magazine subscription. I couldn't detect any feeling in what she was saying. If I were to give that news to someone, I'd be screaming into the phone, "Holy hell, a match! We found a match!" but not Roseann. She was a stone. There was more to the story.

My match was a woman in her sixties from California. Roseann explained that the woman was highly sensitized, which meant she was a match for me, but her body had developed antibodies that may fight off my kidney.[42] She didn't tell me any more about her other than she had a donor in her life that would also give a kidney to someone else, and a chain would commence. Roseann said I should think about it, talk with Mat, and then call her back. I could choose to decline this recipient if this were a risk I did not want to take.

What I heard from our phone exchange was that if I chose to donate to this woman, there was a good chance my kidney would die. It was more complicated than that, involving science, drugs, technology, and big words. My kidney may live a short time and extend her life, but it would most likely die. That is what I took away from our conversation. My kidney would die trying to save that woman in California.

The grief I felt about turning her down still sneaks up on me, even today. At the time, she was around the same age as my dad's wife, Kay, whom I adored. If Kay needed a kidney and was "highly sensitized," would I have made the same decision? I don't know, maybe. In a sense, I had denied Kay, by way of this unknown woman, a longer life because of my fear of her antibodies killing my kidney off. That guilt has been hard to shake.

I wanted my kidney to have a long life, and I also liked the idea of others having a little skin in the game by way of their family members donating to strangers, too. Perhaps I couldn't have both in this system. Perhaps I had to accept that not everything would unfold as neatly as I had expected. My kidney may die, but other kidneys in the chain could live on. My kidney could live, but others in the chain could die. Was the reassurance that at least someone lived on because of my efforts enough? Did the outcome really have to be perfect?

Weeks passed without communication from Loyola, and life went on. Mat and I committed to two New Year's resolutions of becoming vegetarians and running some sort of race. I spent a few days every week barely at a jog on our old country road, getting ready for race day, which we hadn't even chosen. Still, whenever we did pick the race and the day to stand at the starting line, I didn't want to fall behind. As impossible as it sounded, I wanted us to run it together.

We continued our renovations of the house, rebuilding a porch on the front and painting a couple of bedrooms. I helped plan the commemoration of the Memorial Day Massacre in Chicago; I was in Detroit for the Steelworkers' Rapid Response Convention; I made 600 ham sandwiches for volunteers at the United Way Day of Caring, all the while wondering how hard it was to be rematched. Maybe the woman from California was my only match, and I blew my chance to help someone, simply out of fear.

By this time, I had been getting mail from Loyola every week, and not the good kind. Like most giant systems with lots of data, codes, and processes, the Loyola billing system was not aligned with the Loyola transplant center. They were unaware that I would never be liable to pay them for any services, so they kept reminding me of what I owed. My thyroid ultrasound bill was $576. Then, it was adjusted down to $299, and another bill was sent. Then they reminded me that I still owed them $299. Then, they reminded me again.

As I looped in the transplant center to intervene, the bills continued to come. I ignored it all, hoping it would be handled appropriately without me, until I received a letter saying I was being sent to collections. A steam cloud appeared from the top of my head, just like in the cartoons. I prided myself on paying my debts, and my credit was flawless. But there I was, being pulled into collections because of a billing system that had not kept pace with the times. I did my best to be cordial with the collection agency and the Loyola staff, but I'm sure it was obvious how frustrated that made me. A billing experience like this could deter potential donors, and there weren't enough of us to leave that to chance.

It was early in May that Roseann called. She needed me to draw more blood and would send the tubes through the mail again. Roseann didn't tell me any more than that. The package Loyola sent had the same instructions as the last time: fill the vials, put them in the box, and send them the bill. But this time, there were two differences. There were twice as many vials, and they were being mailed to two different locations.

I looked up Pinnacle Health System, the second place my blood was to be mailed to. It was in Pennsylvania. Pinnacle wasn't an affiliate of Loyola but instead another medical center. Either Loyola needed help from an outside lab, or someone in Pennsylvania had their eye on my kidney. Regardless, it wouldn't be the first time my DNA traveled to the Keystone State.

For much of 2008, I lived in the Lawrenceville neighborhood, a hub of great coffee and working-class families in Pittsburgh. The Steelworkers International Union brought me on as a technician in its Strategic Campaigns Department at its downtown headquarters. It was an opportunity to be hired full-time with my union eventually. Since it was a contingent role at first, Mat stayed in Indiana to work, and I moved without him, experiencing what Pittsburgh had to offer all on my own.

Pittsburgh had a big city feel, but was easy to navigate once I got my highly complicated first-ever public transit experience out of the way. The people were friendly, and my friends Jason and Liz, who were moving away, allowed me to live in their home as a trial run. I wondered if there was someone in that region who needed my kidney.

Did I sit next to them on my many bus rides? How wild would it be if they were one of my neighbors or coworkers? Maybe I passed them on the toll road.

Less than a year after arriving in the city, the Great Recession caused me to pack my bags and head home. It also caused Mat to lose his job the day after I did. But that's a story for another book, perhaps—working-class angst in a world of plenty. My time in Pittsburgh was limited by a nation in turmoil, but the possibility that I was in the same city as someone who would need me years later was bonkers to imagine.

It didn't take long for Roseann to call me back after my blood was shipped out. Another match had been found. She again couldn't tell me much about the person, other than it was a man from Pennsylvania, and he had a donor in his life who would also give away a kidney to someone else. If he were "highly sensitized," Roseann didn't say, and I was hesitant to ask.

I wondered whether they had to tell you those things because of policy or just as a matter of courtesy, so I could make an informed decision. If a potential donor knows too many details about a potential recipient, this process could boil down to more than just a goodwill gesture from one person to another. It could be unethical, and I understood that.

I was excited that a second match had been found for me. But at the same time, I felt completely sapped. It was already May 2012. My life was booked solid for the next few months with classes, conventions, and workshops. My obligations to my work were important to me, but now a real-life person was depending on me, too—a person waiting on me to throw him a lifeline.

Roseann said I could choose the date for surgery, and everyone would work around me to make sure I was able to fulfill all my obligations. Mat and I looked through the calendar to see when we could both be free at the same time. The end of July was our first window. It was our anniversary week. He agreed to tend to my post-surgery needs as we celebrated our twelfth year of marriage.

We set July 26th for the big day. The exact time and details would come as the date drew nearer. Roseann asked that I stay in the area the week after surgery to be nearby if there were any complications. Plus, a post-surgery follow-up appointment with Dr. Milner would be necessary at the end of that week, which I'd need to be available for. Diane from NKR would handle all of those arrangements for us.

So, it was officially official. I had been medically cleared to donate a kidney. I had a person in Pennsylvania who would be receiving it. I had a husband who was completely majestic and fully supportive of my decision. Now there was only one thing left to do: I had to tell people.

Mat and I split up the responsibility of informing our families of the details. He told his family, and I told mine. Mat's immediate family had good questions, and he answered them well. A lot of head shaking commenced between them, simply out of curiosity. The news spread throughout his bloodline by word of mouth after that. I didn't have to answer questions or explain myself. Instead, I had to endure that look when I saw them—that genuine look of wonderment.

Dad, again, showed zero interest in hearing anything about my surgery, even though he listened intently as I told Kay about the impending date. As usual, his eyes were focused on the screen of the TV, while his ears were tuned into the perimeter of the room. I think he really did want to know what was happening with the surgery, without acknowledging as much. I was 35, a full-grown adult person at that time. Regardless of anyone's objections, I was going to do what I was moved to do.

My sister had good questions, but was relatively low-key about the whole thing, too. I asked her to tell the kids, and she wondered if she should tell them at all. For a minute, I wondered along with her. If I did not plan to tell the world, did the kids need to know? Still, I wanted them to learn ahead of surgery what Aunt Rae had up her sleeve. It was one of those "teachable moments" Oprah always talked so fondly about. The kids could heed a lesson from this family story. Maybe that was Dara's apprehension; perhaps she couldn't explain it. It was even hard for me to explain, and I was doing the thing. My surgery wasn't intended for headline news, but I wanted those close to me to know about it.

By the end of May, my core squad knew. I consistently worked with a small cadre of dedicated people. They needed to know because they were with me on a daily basis via calls, videos, or in-person meetings. We collaborated on events and developed training programs together, and became very close through the years, and I considered them like family. Everyone else I interacted with was still unaware of my impending surgery. It was hard enough for me to talk about it with those who were close to me. To tell the world would feel much too flashy for my style.

Chapter 9

# If I Only Had More Spares

We had two months of living to get done before the July 26th surgery, and I was busier than ever. Not only was I attending the Indiana Republican Party Convention to speak about Hoosier manufacturing and trade, but I also had double duty for the state Democratic Party Convention. Congressional District Chairperson for the Democratic Party, Carmen Darland, enlisted my help in planning a first-of-its-kind expo for regional manufacturing companies to market their products to the public. Supporting manufacturing was, obviously, at the core of my occupation, so it was a great project to organize. By the time the dust settled, the exhibitors at the Northeast Indiana Manufacturing Showcase had filled the historic two-story Embassy Theater adjoining the convention hall with pickles and pick-up trucks, tires and candy. It was grand.

The Indiana Alliance for Retired Americans, which is always a lovely collection of Hoosier retirees from multiple industries, had me speak on trade and jobs at their annual convention in Indianapolis. I traveled to DC for the Good Jobs Green Jobs Conference and corresponding advocacy work with Congress. My time off the clock was minimal during this period because justice rarely gets a day off, ya know. I was with many of my colleagues in the months leading up to my surgery, but I never brought up my kidney relocation. There was too much work to be done for anyone's attention to be turned awkwardly toward me.

During the first part of July, Diane reached out to see how Mat and I were feeling. Were we excited? Did we have any questions? My annual advocacy workshop for steelworkers at the University of

Illinois was the week before surgery, from Sunday through Friday, July 15 – 20. That week had always been very busy for me, so we asked her all of the questions we had to prevent any last-minute revelations.

I shared an NPR article on donors with Diane.[43] It was published just a few weeks prior and had a few scary bits of news, most notably that kidney donors weren't treated very well. The article featured two donors who developed health problems after their surgeries that were either not disclosed to them as potential risks by their transplant centers or that they did not financially plan for.

The article explained the details of an insurance policy the Living Organ Donor Network spearheaded to protect donors. It was meant to be a tool for peace of mind and would help donors with residual medical expenses related to surgery in the event they developed complications. It also had a life insurance component if a donor were to die because of the donation. However, just six of the 260 transplant centers across the country had their donors enrolled in it. Bringing up the downside, they concluded, could scare people away from donating.

My question to Diane was simple: Do I get this insurance? The article didn't make me apprehensive about the surgery, but it did make me want to get in on any programs that could help me if I needed them. Even though it was a highly unlikely scenario, the article made me want to have that kind of protection in case it all went south. Diane said NKR covered the $500 policy cost for each of its donors, and I would receive paperwork to complete for it soon.

As a donor herself, Diane had a lot of solid experience to share. After surgery, I would feel fatigued. I'd have an incision on my stomach, so I shouldn't lift more than ten pounds for a while. I shouldn't use NSAID pain relievers like aspirin or ibuprofen, just Tylenol or whatever they provided at the hospital. Drawstring pants and button-down shirts were recommended to keep my clothes from being tight around my waist. Pillows to protect my stomach from the seat belt for the ride home should also be included in our packing list.

Movement was important, in more ways than one, Diane noted. The more I could be up and out of bed after surgery, the better I'd feel. The staff would do whatever was necessary to make sure my bowels were working properly before I would be discharged. In other words, I couldn't leave Loyola until I passed gas and made sure they knew about it.

The anesthesia would paralyze my intestines so much so that it would take seven to ten days for the entire length of it to get back to work. The thought of having ten days of food inside me waiting for the "train to leave the station" was frightening. I could not imagine how so many days of digested food would feel waiting for its turn to exit.

Since I didn't know any of the surgery details, Diane gave me Roseann's direct line. For Diane to book my hotel for the correct days after surgery, she needed to know, too. My task was to reach out to Roseann to get answers about surgery specifics, my NLDAC paperwork (which we began in November for financial assistance), and the name of my Donor Advocate, and then circle back with Diane.

When Roseann, Mat, and I finally spoke on July 12, I believe we both left that conversation flustered with a side order of frustration. We had set the surgery date for July 26, two months ahead of time, because I would be unavailable and out of town working until then. Roseanne explained that I needed more lab work the week before my surgery, which was never mentioned in my schedule of events. After numerous phone calls and emails, Roseann identified a lab near the University and arranged for them to handle my blood work. Their hours would enable me to get my blood drawn before my workshop began. That was an amenable compromise. A workaround was the only option, and Roseann surely found it.

It seemed a lot had changed in my status since I last spoke with any Loyola folks. We had gone from "be patient" to "hurry-the-hell-up" mode in very little time. My social worker had been Janice, but now I was assigned to Kaitlin. Since my application for NLDAC funding began with Janice in 2011, I had to start the paperwork again with Kaitlin using 2012 information about my updated household income and W-2s. Kaitlin reached out to ask me to complete all the paperwork and send it back to her the very next day.

My donor advocate, who may have also been Janice at one time, had been changed to Dr. Vavra, the doctor who checked my thyroid in October. He would reach out to me soon. Roseann explained that my surgery would be early on Thursday morning, and I would be admitted into the hospital the day before, on the 25th. That way, our three-or four-hour drive from Auburn to Maywood could be done without the fear of running late to my very own surgery.

The NLDAC form was four pages long. I was able to complete it that evening and send it back to Kaitlin along with our pay stubs showing our income. The line on the form that gave me the option to explain my connection to the recipient had to be checked off as "other" because the only options were blood or family choices like "Mother" or "Spouse."

I had to attest that there was no "valuable consideration" being exchanged for my kidney. No one was buying my kidney from me— not for cash, not for a cruise around the world, or a Randy "Macho Man" Savage collectible figurine. My signature on the dotted line declared I wasn't in it for the money.

At the end of the form were four true or false statements that I needed to answer to determine the need for funding programs like it to exist:

The NLDAC will make it possible for me to donate an organ.

The NLDAC program will help reduce my stress and give me less worry.

I had hoped that the recipient would have received a deceased donor organ.

I wish that NLDAC could assist with lost pay or vacation/leave.

They all sounded like trick questions. If I were able to donate an organ without NLDAC funding, should I mark that statement as true anyway, so I didn't jeopardize the program for those who couldn't afford it? But if I marked it as true and didn't get the funding, would that signal to them that I couldn't afford to go through with the surgery, and they would call the whole thing off? I just closed my eyes and filled in a circle.

The Living Organ Donor Network insurance form was five pages long. There was a box to check that identified my recipient and me without labeling me as an "other": "Altruistic, random recipient."

My employer benefits had to be explained, including our household income and how much of it was attributed to my wages. Then, there were questions about my surgery. Questions I must have been expected to know:

What type of procedure will you have?

Laparoscopic? Open Incision? Unknown?

Which kidney do you anticipate being used for your donation?

Left? Right? Unknown?

If I guessed at this, I had a 50% chance of being right. I had no idea what the correct answer was for either of them. Since it was a life and health insurance policy, it wasn't clear to me why the questions were even relevant. If donating one kidney or another offered more of a risk to my life, the doctors would choose wisely, right?

That weekend, I was working in the garden, finishing some final weeding before my bending and stretching would be limited by a bloated stomach, when Dad walked over from next door and said he wanted to talk to me about my surgery. "You're doing alright with two, you should keep two," he said. For Dad to offer one last plea for me to cancel the surgery was admirable. He knew, deep down in his gut, that I was not changing my mind. Still, he tried one more time. That's what dads do, I suppose.

"I am not going to let that guy down, Dad."

My time in Illinois, working with steelworkers from District 7, and my corresponding blood draw near the university went off without a hitch. It was a fruitful week of doing what I enjoyed, surrounded by hardworking Midwestern union members. Two hundred of my people were there, but just one, my co-facilitator pal Tom, knew what was on my agenda for the very next week, and he kept it all to himself.

Back at home that Sunday, I was surprised by a family ambush. Mat's dad and Ruth stopped by with a stockpile of strawberry shortcake and homemade ice cream. Soon after, relatives were coming up the driveway and pouring in the doors. Nieces, nephews, sisters and brothers, Mat's mom, and even Dad and Kay came over. They all sat around our big dining room table and celebrated this thing I was about to do, while I awkwardly visited and tried not to talk about the thing they were all there to talk about.

Ruth had asked Mat about coming out to see me off before the big day, and he conveniently didn't mention it until after they all showed up. It was a very kind gesture, but it made me terribly uneasy. Attention like that wasn't a comfortable space to live in for me. The cards and the drawings the kids made for me were so sweet, but I couldn't look at any of them until everyone left, for I'd surely be a puddle of tears. That sort of involuntary response would contradict the very composed and straight-faced persona I had worked my whole life to perfect.

Later that evening, I scanned the $46 receipt I had for the blood draw near the university. I added it to an email directed to all the addresses I had for the Loyola staff I'd communicated with over the past year and a half. In the email were the questions I declared to be my last and final before doing this thing. My first question was, where am I supposed to go on Wednesday?

Joanna reached out on Monday, and we were able to get into the details. Roseann, with whom I had been communicating the most, would be out of the office for a few weeks. Joanna was now the answerer of questions. She sent me precise information on where to be and when:

***Wednesday, July 25, 2012 - Please arrive at the Main Hospital Admitting Area, Room 1101, at 1:00 p.m.*** *You will be admitted to a floor unit once a room is available, where you will have your blood drawn, a urine test, and you will meet with the transplant surgery team to sign surgical consents and also meet with an anesthesiologist.*

***Thursday, July 26, 2012 - Your surgery is planned to begin around 5:00 a.m.*** *You will be taken down to the Pre-Operative holding area probably between 3:30 a.m. and 4:00 a.m.; please make sure that any visitors or family who may want to see you do so beforehand. You probably will not be back onto the floor in your room until late morning or early afternoon.*

Joanna also updated me on the status of my NLDAC application.

I did not qualify for assistance from the government program because my application was incomplete. The income of my recipient needed to be factored into the equation to process my paperwork, but there wasn't enough time to get it. Plus, we, as a household, made too much money. This was indeed a strange program. To connect the incomes of anyone, much less complete strangers, in this way seemed like a clunky system in need of an overhaul, or at least a revision.

As for food, Joanna suggested I eat light on Wednesday before being admitted. They would have me on an IV that night, and I would not be allowed to eat after that. She also reminded me not to take NSAIDs that week or for the following six months.

I updated Diane on the conversation with Joanna about NLDAC, and she said NKR would reimburse me for any meal and travel expenses for the trip, Mat included. So, because NDLAC declined my application, NKR made sure it would not cost us any money to donate my kidney. I just needed to keep a record and send the receipts to Diane as I had done before.

Mat and I went on a last-minute supply run, including a trip to Big Lots for packets of oatmeal and canned soups. That store always had deals on organic, vegetarian food. NKR was picking up the tab for our expenses, but we weren't going to step outside of our typical frugal protocol. The lower our expenses, the better able NKR would be to pay for the next donor's meals.

On our way home that day, we stopped at the union hall for the local BF Goodrich tire plant, USW Local 715L. I needed to drop off some last-minute paperwork to my pal Herb. We had a monthly Central Labor Council meeting that I was going to miss because of my surgery, and I needed to let him know. In twenty words or less I told him why. He was surprised but didn't bombard me with questions. He simply wished me well.

The days and weeks leading up to the surgery didn't feel like anything out of the ordinary for me. My senses weren't heightened. I didn't have contradicting thoughts running through my head, despite Dad's last and final plea. There was no second-guessing myself. I had the surgery marked on my pocket calendar just like any other agenda item.

This was something I wanted to do, and then I was going to celebrate my sister-in-law Mollie's wedding. Then, I was going to write that editorial about the Indiana automotive industry. After that, I had the Labor Day Picnic to set up for. Then I was going to figure out which race Mat and I would run before 2012 came to an end.

I had become an agenda-driven kind of person. The things I want to do, I do. Then, I move on to do other things I want to do. There is no need to mull things over for an eternity before taking a plunge. Nope, no regrets here. I plan things out, and then I do them. Right or wrong, as the head architect, that is how I designed my life. That is how I feel useful and productive, by doing and experiencing as much as I can as often as I can. Maybe I don't stop to ponder insignificant things or smell the roses as often as the average person, but flowers die, and I have the world to explore.

Mat didn't have any last-minute doubts about the surgery either. If he did, he didn't share them with me. We were partners in all things wild and crazy or ordinary and boring. I knew I was fortunate to have him by my side during that time. He was the only one who could have changed my mind. Instead, he chose to go with my gut and follow my lead.

Our road trip to Maywood took a typical pit stop for us, a visit to Rise and Roll. It was a bakery in the heart of Middlebury, an Amish community along Highway 20. Their motto was "Life is Short, Eat Dessert First," and they had the display cases to back that up: bacon-wrapped maple donuts, lemon-filled powdered donuts, and traditional glazed. I would often stop there on my road trips for work to use the restroom, but also to grab snacks of the healthier persuasion.

Surgery would begin at 5 a.m. the next morning. Why anyone would voluntarily get up that early in the morning is beyond me, but I wanted to give Dr. Milner a little fuel for the long day ahead. Our gift of choice: Veggie Stix. They had the consistency of Pringles, were shaped like carrot sticks, and were full of air like cheese curls. Made with flour from various vegetables, they had become a favorite of ours in our mission to become healthy vegetarians, one of our 2012 New Year's resolutions.

We documented the trip with photos. Our first one was of me in front of the Rise and Roll. It marked the last time both of my kidneys would pee in that building. Before being admitted that afternoon, Mat and I went to the Loyola cafeteria. Our second photo taken was of my kidneys having their "last supper" together there. From the candy-striper days of my youth, I had always been a fan of hospital food. You could always find something healthy or greasy on the buffet, depending on your mood. That day, potato soup and a giant salad were my choice. It was an honorable meal to end my beloved relationship with my kidney.

Upon checking into the hospital, we were escorted to our room. It reminded me of the maternity ward in our local hospital. Mat and I had made multiple visits to that floor to welcome babies into our family. Our room was big enough for a family of ten awaiting the arrival of a new little person. The couch along the wall by the window turned into a bed. Our bags and laptops fit perfectly in the cabinets on either side of the couch, and we had our own bathroom and shower. They made sure we were comfortable.

It wasn't long before we were in full hospital action mode. The nurses and aides assigned to work with me were: Annie, Megan, Jen, Deepa, Anna, Miranda, Jeanette, Meredith, and Merlita. All came in when their shifts began, introduced themselves, and got to work. Blood draws and urine tests commenced. The anesthesiologist came in with questions. A doctor of this and a doctor of that also stopped to check in. I had my hospital gown on and green slipper socks out of the bag before our suitcase was even unpacked. We were moving right along.

Soon after, Dr. Milner walked in, bringing with him a string of medical students with note pads and pens. He was full of the same brand of happiness I remembered from October. I'd guess he was high-spirited to be in his natural habitat, doing the work of connecting the kidney dots. He shared the details of how the following day would transpire. It would be an early one, but I'd be done and awake by the afternoon.

The students, all in their own white coats and shiny shoes, were taking notes as Dr. Milner talked to Mat and me. They peered up from their words now and then, like they were recording the movements of a rare endangered species in the wild. I'd smile if one caught my eye, but they'd quickly drop their focus back to the pages, concentrating on their discoveries. It must have been an exciting moment for them to witness something good come from a hospital stay.

Dr. Milner informed us that we may have a wrench thrown into our chain. He didn't want me to worry, but there was weather a'coming. A storm was predicted over Pennsylvania at the same time as my kidney was scheduled to fly there. If flights were canceled or delayed, my kidney might not be able to get to its intended recipient. Thankfully, there was a Plan B.

Two people in the vicinity of Loyola were on standby. Both needed a kidney, and each of them could do just fine with mine. They were instructed to wait nearby in case my kidney's plane couldn't take off. In case Mother Nature caused my recipient to lose his chance, one of them would be called upon and gladly accept it.

Imagine that. Two people in desperate need of a kidney, waiting for another person, also in need of a kidney, to be passed up by the weather. Three people were patiently waiting on the other end of my one organ, and that Pennsylvania weather left everyone in suspense. I can't fully grasp how that must have felt to be the two people nearby, waiting for our plan to backfire. How overjoyed one of them would have been to receive my kidney. How sad it would be for them to know it was because someone else was just too far away.

I was glad Dr. Milner and his team were prepared enough that if my kidney couldn't find its way to its perfect match, it wouldn't go to waste. I was also glad that it wouldn't just be sewn back into me, good as new, after we'd gone through all of the work to get here. There would indeed be a recipient.

Dr. Milner said his goodbyes, and his entourage of students went with him. Mat and I settled into our room, unpacked the bag, and checked in with family. By 5:30, a plate of liquid food was delivered to me. Cups of broth, apple juice, sherbet, and ice filled the tray. Confused, I checked in with the nurse about my eating restrictions. She said I didn't have any. My "last supper" picture was retaken to reflect my official last supper for both of my kidneys together.

A student or two would come and go through our room, looking at my chart or taking my vitals. They'd almost tiptoe so they didn't disturb me. I was curious about them. Were they going to become kidney surgeons like Dr. Milner? Were they almost finished with school? I'd smile and try to engage, but that was not within the confines of our relationship. They'd stiffen up, smile, and leave the room. Mat told me to leave them alone to focus on their work, but I can't help but work the room, no matter the room.

Mat eventually left to find his own dinner in the cafeteria, which gave me time to breathe and take in the space. It was a big room for little old me. Nothing major was happening in this room to need so much space. We could have done just fine in one half its size, but maybe that was the Red-Carpet treatment Loyola patients received all the time. Embrace the pampering, I suppose.

My pal Mike called, but when I answered the phone, we were on a full-blown conference call "Hospital-Style" with our friends Mick, Meghan, and Kenny. It was heartwarming to hear the voices of the people with whom I had worked so closely over the past few years. To hear their kind words of appreciation and love for me and their well-wishes for a speedy recovery meant a lot. They were rooting for me, and they knew it was hard for me to verbalize how much I appreciated them. Still, they had no problem finding the words.

By 7:30, Mat was back in our room with me, and we were greeted with yet another food delivery. My new tray contained salad, cottage cheese, bread, soup, and a piece of vanilla cake. It was my third "last supper," which warranted yet another picture. In the back of my mind, I was thinking about how long all that food would be cooped up in my system. My body would have no interest in a bathroom break before my 3:30 a.m. wake-up call for surgery. That meant it was with me for the long haul. Seven to ten days, they said. It'd be fine, they said.

The papers I signed that day were hefty. The words were big. The meanings were even bigger. The first was a "Consent to Treat" document with standard language about payments and responsibilities. It was a form likely signed by everyone, whether they were liable to pay for their own care or not. It stated that I was responsible for paying Loyola for services rendered. In reality, I wasn't.

The eight-page "Informed Consent to Donate a Kidney for Transplantation" handout felt very much like a last-chance cautionary tale. It was a parent informing their child of impending doom if they ran across the street. Even though the ice-cream truck is just on the other side, and there are puppies and a Ferris wheel, if you run across that street, you could get hit by a car. You could trip and scuff your knee. You could get to the ice-cream truck, and there might be none left. The ice cream truck could evaporate into thin air before you make it to the other side.

The document was designed to make me ask: Do I really want to run across the street for ice cream? Am I prepared if I scuff my knee? I could always eat the Push-Ups in the freezer instead. Did I consider that option? Who likes ice cream anyway?

Center-specific outcomes were listed, comparing Loyola's survival rates with the national average. There was a section emphasizing that I could change my mind at any time during the process. And then, another gentle reminder that insurance companies might not find me attractive after this whole debacle. My premiums may increase; they may not pay for medical care I would need, and my lack of a kidney could be a pre-existing condition to warrant my full and complete expulsion from their policies.

All of this was meant to steer anyone with the least little bit of apprehension away from the operating table. The risks, the consequences, and the lifelong decision I was making were clearly not for everyone. It could not be undone. Once the anesthesia was pumped in, there was no going back. Was I sure I wanted to do this? Really? Do you want to think about it some more? Still sure? How about now?

I appreciated all the caution around the decision. Considering that at one time the medical community thought non-directed donors had mental illness for even wanting to help a stranger in that way, I was glad they had come far enough along to give us the green light at all. I had successfully reached this point, and twenty-one months later, there ain't no going back.

It was 10:30 p.m., and Mat and I were still snapping pictures. He had always been such a solid supporter of me and my ideas and goals. In all things, he was my number one fan. He looked calm and at ease, but I still wondered if he, like Dad, was harboring fear of what might come. I hoped I wasn't putting him through that kind of hell. I hoped he knew I didn't mean for him to bear any burden, other than to hold my hand through awesome times such as these, just as I would for him.

It was midnight when the nurse came in to wake me. In her hand was yet another cup. It was the final time both of my kidneys peed together, all for a last-minute pregnancy test. I looked over at Mat, sound asleep on the couch ten feet away. I always knew we'd do great things together in life. If we had each other, boundaries would cease to exist. He had to realize just how awesome I thought he was, but it never hurts to make it official.

I tucked it away in a spot he'd have to eventually find: in the desk drawer, inside the checkbook. In my mind, everything would be fine, but just in case my intuition had let me down in a major way, he needed to know how I felt about my life with him. Plus, he needed a road map to where the important files were.

Written on a sheet of our factory letterhead, I told him how much richer my life had been for having him in it. It was full of sweetness, coupled with instructions on what bills needed to be paid, for I'd hate it if he had to spend any amount of time searching for what I could easily identify for him. I folded the note into a loose piece of paper from my desk, the Digest of Senate Bill 401. That public works bill had been one of a myriad of projects I was tackling to help working people in Indiana. Why I chose to wrap my love for Mat around that legislation, I don't recall. I'm just glad he never needed to read it.

# Chapter 10

# Me and the Guy Down the Hall

I asked Mat what he remembered of the big day seven years after it happened. His memory, I thought, would be a lot clearer than mine and would help me illuminate this chapter. My recollection was strong, but I was sedated and in and out of sleep. Surely, he had tidbits of time stored away in his mind that I wasn't awake to experience.

"I have a lousy memory for that, babe. I don't even remember meeting Dr. Milner until we saw him in New York. Movie quotes from 20 years ago, sure, but not what happened on July 26, 2012."

In this chapter, you get my recollection as far as I and the morphine know it to be true.

From what I could tell, I hadn't even entered REM sleep before the staff started piling in. Hearing the movements, I opened my eyes to see multiple smiling faces standing over me. Then Mat appeared, sleepy but also smiling. It was time. A boulder appeared out of nowhere in my throat, just seeing his smile.

If I had a chance to wash my face or brush my teeth, I don't recall. Was my hair disheveled? Did I have to pee? The minutes I was awake that morning were a complete blur. A person dressed in surgical clothes asked if I was ready. I shook my head. Mat bent down to kiss me, tell me he loved me, and that he would see me soon.

The bed started moving as the blue-cloaked angels all took their places alongside me to do the pushing. My world was silent. No beeping of machines or voices over the speakers could be heard. The lights along the hallways were dim. I didn't have any expectations for how that moment would play out. That may have been how all donors were transported to surgery. Quiet, dark halls offer time to reflect one last time before the knife appears. Someone hovered over me and said he was giving me something to sleep. I nodded my head, and seconds later, I disappeared into the darkness.

What happened next, I can only presume to be magic. While I was fully present yet entirely unaware, that operating room, piled high with surgeons, nurses, anesthesiologists, and aides, collectively revealed how a simple act of generosity could help heal the world in a small but very big way. Together, we all did a thing that would have been forbidden a decade before: we dared to care about a perfect stranger.

It was many hours later when I opened my eyes again. I woke up in a post-operative recovery area. My body felt heavy, and my head felt equally weighted. Mat was sitting in the chair next to me. His smile partially masked his concern as he told me everything went well. Then, I closed my eyes.

Finally, I woke up in my original hospital room. Mat was sitting on the couch across from my bed, talking to Dad on the phone. Gently, I felt around my stomach. My hand was touching my body, but I couldn't feel it. It must have been the meds. Much like getting a cavity filled, if you eat before the Novocain subsides, you won't be able to tell that you just chewed half your cheek off.

I was curious to see what happened to my body. As I tried to pull the covers down and my gown up, Mat stood up to stop me. There were wires and tubes all over, and he was afraid I'd disconnect something important. Connected to me was a heart monitor, a catheter, and an IV. At the end of the bed, I also had a machine that squeezed my legs like a blood pressure cuff every now and then. I was fully loaded with all the bells and whistles. Mat helped navigate the connections so that I could see Dr. Milner's handiwork.

My stomach, with its new holes and puffiness, was yellow, having been doused with iodine. There were dots and lines and numbers written on my stomach with a marker as if it were a map leading to a buried treasure. I had four one-inch slits on the left side of my navel with what looked like pieces of scotch tape covering them. Then, about six inches south of my navel, I saw a four-inch horizontal slice of redness, also being held together by scotch tape. There weren't staples or stitches to be found anywhere. Instead, medical-grade glue sealed my incisions, with tape as backup.

At my request, Mat took pictures of my bloated, yellow stomach. Looking half-baked, I gave the peace sign as he snapped a shot of me lying in bed. I didn't realize how far south the horizontal incision was until he pointed it out. To the naked, unmedicated eye, that incision was about as low as it could go.

People were coming in and out of our room, checking my vitals, checking in. I just lay there, my mind in a state of disarray. I wanted to go back to sleep, but I also wanted to know which one made it to Pennsylvania: the storm or my kidney.

Eventually, Dr. Milner came in to assess me. He told us what we already knew: the surgery went perfectly. As he checked my vitals, he informed us that my kidney had indeed arrived in Pennsylvania, safe and sound, after all. I didn't ask, but I wondered how the other two local people waiting in the wings for my kidney took that news. Our dance with Mother Nature had come and gone, leaving both of them back on the dreaded transplant waitlist.

Mat was on duty as our receptionist, answering our phones, my work phone, and the phone in the room, as family and friends called to check in on us. My friend Mike was the first to call. When I got on the phone, it was yet another group conference call with my pals. I'm sure it was comical for them to hear me fully medicated, trying to form sentences.

As the staff praised my urine collection at the end of my catheter, they encouraged me to drink. All the water and ice I wanted were at my disposal, so I could continue filling the bag. I suppose, the day a kidney is removed, and one is left behind, it's important to be sure it's picking up the slack and can "carry the water," so to speak.

Dr. Milner soon returned, this time bearing gifts. He pulled his phone out of his pocket and fidgeted a bit before showing Mat and me the screen. We saw a man in a hospital gown. The lighting in his room was behind him, making his image look more like a shadow than a fully defined person. He was wearing glasses and lying in a bed, speaking into the camera. We could see all of this, but could hear absolutely nothing. Mat and I looked at Dr. Milner, confused.

As he turned the phone back toward himself to try to figure out the volume problem, my first hunch was that the man was my recipient and that the video had come straight from Pennsylvania as a special delivery. But what was he saying?

Finally, Dr. Milner, defeated, apologized for being all thumbs with his new phone, turned the video back to me, and said, "This is the guy down the hall. He's thanking you for saving his life."

I didn't even know there WAS a "guy down the hall." And, what was he doing thanking ME? As Dr. Milner explained, our eyes leaked everywhere. My kidney was most definitely in Pennsylvania, but someone in that man's life gave one away, too. We knew that was going to happen, but we did not know that THAT kidney was now officially… officially, inside "the guy down the hall." Two planes took flight on July 26, 2012. My kidney went to Pennsylvania, and another person's kidney came right back, to begin and end a chain of four.

I continued to sip whatever liquids the staff brought me, but soon felt nauseous. Each time I had any amount of liquid going in, it would come right back out in my bedpan. My stomach felt so heavy and chill on the outside, yet on the inside, an aggressive revolution had been declared against hydration. I didn't feel a thing, except the need to puke.

The staff had Dr. Milner return to check on me. He suspected my nausea was a reaction to the anesthesia. It is hard to guess how someone will react to something until they've experienced it. That was my first major surgery, and as far as my memory could claim, my first major dose of anesthesia. I guessed that the consequence wasn't anything we could have prevented. I had to push through it. I would get fluids from the IV until the nausea subsided. In the meantime, I drank it down and threw it up.

As the night wound down and the traffic in our room dwindled, I got on the phone with Dad and Kay, and then my sister. I was still heavily medicated, but I remember singing to them. It was my way of showing them that I was just fine, and all that worry was for nothing. However, my slurry disposition may have given them the opposite impression. Either way, we were on the other side of my decision. My kidney was gone, and there was no turning back.

The next day, I was scheduled to be released from the hospital to move into our hotel room down the street. Since I was still unable to keep anything down, they decided to keep me there. That was fine. What's another day of hospital pampering while I puke my guts out?

As I was heaving over the side of the bed, my pal Mike tiptoed in. He lived less than an hour from Loyola and wanted to check in on me. We were close enough that I was pleased to see him, even at my worst. Horrified at the sight of me filling up the bedpan, he quickly placed a card on the table, said he'd return later, and walked backward out of the room. I can't say I blamed him. I didn't look so good.

Friends and family continued to check in throughout the day. All of them spoke in a low, peculiar whisper. I thought the morphine was distorting my reality, but no, everyone talked as if not to wake the baby. As if they were entering a library and were trying to prevent being shushed. Then I also began whispering as I carried on conversations. We were all whispering. Why were we whispering? Is this a side effect after surgery?

As the medical students gently circled the bed and took their notes, I felt like a full-fledged unicorn: a magical creature in the forest, rarely seen by the naked eye. The students side-eyed me. They politely smiled, pens constantly in motion. Witnessing joy in a hospital must feel really good. Watching over those who played a role in such happy moments must be a rewarding experience.

Diane called in. It was a quick call as she just wanted to make sure everything went well and to ask if I needed anything. We told her about our hospital extension and that we'd be at the LaQuinta by the next day, if my nausea improved.

Mat wheeled the IV stand next to me as I walked along the hallway a few times. Getting out of bed helped me regain my energy, and get my innards moving, and it also piqued my curiosity. Ever since Dr. Milner told us there was a "guy down the hall," I wondered if I'd see him on my strolls through the wing. Would I be able to tell who he was? Would he recognize me in some way?

I didn't know what Dr. Milner had told "the guy down the hall" about me. If he knew what I looked like or if he knew my name was unclear. Anyone who looked at me with the least bit of twinkle in their eye, I suspected to be him. The trouble with this logic was that everyone smiled at me in the halls. Was the hospital full of this guy's family members, and they all knew who I was as I walked through the halls? This made it difficult to decipher who may know me versus who was simply a friendly person at the right place at the right time.

By evening, my nausea was in check, and my catheter was out. Broth and ice were staying down, and I was freely peeing on my own. I felt groggy but didn't have any pain since the IV was still working. My stomach felt heavy, and it was poofy, but I was otherwise on the mend.

Mat had been stewing on something for a whole day before he finally shared it with me. He had kept his feelings to himself until he could no longer. He handed me his phone with an email pulled up.

"I almost sent this, but I wasn't sure you wanted the world to know just yet."

Mat had drafted an email addressed to Katie Couric. He told her about me and how much he loved me. He thanked her for her reporting and told her that, because of her, I was in surgery, giving away a kidney. I felt the lump in my throat grow as I read. My husband was hardly a mushy person. Seeing his words to Katie Couric made me so proud of him for writing them. He knew I wanted to keep the surgery on the hush-hush, but his love for me made him come close to spilling the beans.

He was right. I didn't want to tell the world. It would have felt pretentious. Still, I knew I had to accept the fact that all secrets eventually come to light. At that point, half the town, who were all our family, knew of my surgery. It wouldn't be long before the other half learned of it, too.

On Saturday morning, I felt well enough for a shower. I also felt well enough to leave. I had been walking around the halls and back and forth to the restroom without incident. There wasn't much left for me to do to recover other than to rest and to eventually have a bowel movement. Someone else surely needed our hospital room more than we did, and I could recover in the comforts of the hotel.

Dr. Milner came in that afternoon to do one final check on me. Since I was staying nearby, he felt confident about my departure. Any issues I might have in the upcoming week could be resolved with a quick trip back to Loyola. He said he considered having me and "the guy down the hall" meet before I left the hospital, but that they decided against it. He said it may be too soon. He was probably right. It may have been too soon for both of us. I was still groggy and in a bit of a daze. He was, I'm sure, under a good number of drugs too. If I were to meet someone in this chain, I wanted to be ready to meet them with all the jazz hands I could muster.

As Mat and I left the hospital, I met eyes with a dozen people in the halls. Some purposefully smiled my way, others just glanced. I wondered how or if we were connected in a most unusual way. It was a strange feeling to know I had a special connection to someone in the same building I was in, without being able to identify exactly who that person was.

On a daily basis, we pass random people who could be our long-lost cousins or who may someday play a role in our lives. If we saw them today, would we remember that encounter years later? That was some of the allure of doing this, for the wonder that's invoked. We never really know who we're sitting next to on the bus, passing in the hall, or sharing a road with, until we hear their story. And then once we hear it, what are we compelled to do with that information?

Grana, Uncle Ed, Katie Couric, Max Zapata: I'm looking at you…

# Chapter 11

# LaQuinta Inn, A Time for Reflection

LaQuinta Inn is one of those small hotel chains that not everyone knows. It's a tiny outfit, with rooms and service like what you would find at a Holiday Inn: breakfast, laundry, and a pool. My dad and Kay had their wedding reception at the LaQuinta Inn in our town. It's nice enough to celebrate your nuptials without breaking the bank.

I understood why NKR chose that hotel. It served the purpose of helping patients like me recover without the frills of overpriced and unnecessary amenities. It had everything we needed for a week-long stay without a valet, room service, or daily fee for Wi-Fi. Our room was a suite with a lot of the necessities of home: a coffee maker, refrigerator, and microwave.

Mat and I settled in for a week of recovery. From July 28th until my check-up with Dr. Milner on August 1, LaQuinta Inn would be our home. I nestled into the bed and stared hazily at the TV while Mat unpacked and organized the room for our stay. Since he was the IT administrator for our local university, he would be in and out, working a few hours during the week at a nearby satellite campus. He wanted to make sure everything was situated for me so I could easily maneuver around without him.

That evening was the first time in days that I got my computer out and looked through Facebook. It made my heart melt. My sister-in-law, Chandra, posted a cryptic message on my page: "I just wanted to tell you that you are an amazing person!" Then I saw two posts on my page from people I worked with.

It was easy for me to guess how Korene and Carmen found out what I had been up to. I missed a Central Labor Council meeting due to the surgery, and in my absence, my pal Herb from Local 715L spilled the "kidney beans." In a roomful of my union siblings from all over the region, Herb explained why I wasn't there. "The next time you see Rachel Bennett Steury, tell her that she is an amazing person and an inspiration to the community and the world," Carmen wrote. And then Korene, "Thinking of you today. My prayers are with you, too."

The kidney beans would most assuredly be spilled at some point after my surgery, but I didn't know when or how that would transpire, really. It's easy to develop a strategic campaign or an advertising plan for a work event or a petition drive, but a kidney? And could I talk about what I did generally without talking about what I did personally? The idea of tooting one's horn crept into my mind as I debated with myself the virtues of telling one's story against the fact that it would feel self-promoting. That was not within my comfort zone. Telling the world about a surgery in which someone's life was saved, and how the need for more donors is crucial, made sense to me. Telling the world about me and MY surgery, as in "hey look what I did," did not. Why was this such an awkward dilemma for me?

I bet Max Zapata never deliberated with himself the pros and cons of sharing his story with Katie Couric. If he had, I may not have encountered another story like his that would have led me down the path to donation. What would have happened to "the guy down the hall" if that were the case? I bet Garet Hil never second-guessed his need to tell the world, "Kidney donation is awesome; you should try it!" I knew I had to get over the fact that talking about my kidney donation had to include me in the equation, whether I liked it or not.

Many years ago, I had a labor studies class at Indiana University called "Contemporary Labor Problems." In it, a slew of issues unions had been facing, such as automation and international trade, were discussed. But the one issue that really stuck out in my mind was the section about community relations.

Unions were not as effective at building relationships outside of the workplace as they could be. Sometimes they were not highly regarded in their communities because few knew what unions really did or why they were necessary. This was especially true during times of trauma, like during strikes and contract negotiations. The picture painted about unions by management and union-busting law firms was that unions were greedy, money-hungry bastards whose beef was always about money and wanting more of it.

If you're a person IN a union, you typically know better than that. You know a contract negotiation almost always involves disagreements between the company and your union regarding workplace safety, health care, protections for older workers, and wage parity for everyone. You know how much effort you and your union put into your community, and the investment you see all around you is a direct result of the work of the collective. Few people tell that story. Few people hear that story.

Community members, who are often stuck in the middle of these disputes, rarely hear the union's voice, so they are left with half-truths the company spreads. These situations had become such missed opportunities to rally community support that unions rarely reached out to tell the world about the good they did: when they sponsored families for Christmas dinners, when they built houses for the houseless, or when they demanded the company test the drinking water.

Unions were doing tremendous amounts of goodwill, and no one outside the workplace walls knew about it. If no one knew about it, no one could see how essential they were within a workplace, or why they should form one too. Their image problem rested squarely on the fact that they kept their good deeds to themselves. Consequently, workers everywhere feel the effects of decisions like this. Unions need to shout from the rooftops about their goals and their deeds because only through that kind of advocacy can they proclaim why we needed unions in the first place.

I thought about that rationale while lying in that king-sized bed with way too many pillows. Much like unions, I was terrible at talking about myself. Much like unions, I, too, had an important story to tell that could affect the lives of others for years to come. The debate I had with myself shifted from my comfort as a private person to questioning whether that comfort was selfish. Why was I hoarding my story at the expense of people who needed me to tell it?

"It's not about the ship; it's about the cargo."

In my work, I was on one stage or another all the time. I hated being the face of an initiative, but I navigated that road by convincing myself that it wasn't about me; it was about the content I was bringing to the people. It was my voice, but it was never about me. I was safe because there was no need for me to center myself in a presentation about currency manipulation or countervailing duties. The domestic content of a wind turbine or a military bomber did not require anyone staring back at me from their seats to know anything about me. I was the ship.

Alas, the time had come for me to make that distinction in my personal life: I had to be the vessel for the story. As much as I could feel my soul contracting inward at the sheer thought of it, I had to, in whatever way I could, spill the *kidney beans*. I needed to let those words flow out into the universe to help others. I had to let people like "the guy down the hall" know that simple, ordinary people like me existed and to hang on a little longer. I needed to let other people who were curious like me realize they, too, could do something magical for someone else. There was necessary lifesaving organizing work to be done, and I was standing in my own way.

That night, I wrote up a post for Facebook. Since Chandra, Carmen, and Korene had already created a curtain of curiosity, I laid it all on the table for the small group of Facebook friends and family I had at the time. It was my first step in putting myself out there. I put my words in print, not my voice out loud. That, to me, seemed like an agreeable first step to take.

*My Beloved Kidney: Because You Can't [Really] Take it With You...*

I wanted to let my Facebook family know that on Thursday, I went under the knife in Chicago and donated one of my kidneys to someone in Pennsylvania. I started a chain in a "Pay it Forward" program with the National Kidney Registry that helps more sick people get kidneys by having incompatible people in their lives donate kidneys to others who need one. It's all very inspiring, trust me. I only had to watch a segment from Katie Couric to be convinced that it was something I should do. I wanted to send my kidney off in style and let it know I really appreciated all it had done for me for the past 35 years, so I showed it a good time with lots of well water and my favorite red from Satek Winery. On our way to Chicago, we stopped at Rise and Roll and got my transplant crew a mega bag of Veggie Chips, so they were at their best during surgery. I think that did the trick. Veggie chips are like Popeye's spinach, ya know…

Now it's time for my kidney to Cowgirl Up and help this guy in PA. In turn, someone in his life donated a kidney to a guy in Chicago who needed it. He was down the hall from me, getting his new lease on life at Loyola. What a great hospital. I am now recovering, feeling pretty good, but a little sore and tired. I gained 10 pounds of swelling and bloating since Thursday, but that will come off as I get moving around again. My superb Dr. Milner said my kidney function with one kidney is better than that of most people with two kidneys. So… IN YOUR FACE, McDonald's and potato couches! Being active and eating right DOES make the world go 'round. Thank you for all of your thoughts and prayers through the week; it really means a lot to have those positive vibes sent my way. If some of you haven't met my husband, you should know I SCORED BIG with this guy. I couldn't ask for a better husband in this world, with me every step of the way. Love you, baby! It won't be long before I'm back to good, running with the puppies and traveling across the country.

I posted the message, and then I shut the computer down. I didn't want to look, at least not for a while.

For the most part, when I wasn't sleeping, I was lying in bed watching TV. One tidbit of advice I wish I had gotten for my recovery was a clearly prescribed movie restriction. Laughing after you've had your gut cut into produces the same pain as a cough, sneeze, or hiccup, all of which I did that week. The meds dulled the pain, but I still felt it, and it wasn't nice. I learned my lesson the hard way: watch funny movies at your own risk.

Our meals consisted of oatmeal pouches for breakfast and whatever bagel or muffin Mat could grab during the continental breakfast portion of the day. Lunch was an easy can of soup I put in the microwave while Mat was away working. We had bananas, canned fruit, and Veggie Stix on hand for the munchies. For dinners, Mat would get take-out and bring it back, or we would venture out together for some fresh air.

I was getting around fine, albeit slowly and hazily. I felt the urge to hold my stomach often, like pregnant women do to support the weight of a growing belly. It was a strange reflex to develop, but it also felt necessary. My stomach was bloated from the surgery, and it felt like I had a Nerf ball tucked inside. It was a little dense, a little squishy, and a little heavy.

Mat and I celebrated our wedding anniversary during our LaQuinta stay. We had been married for twelve years and together for sixteen by that point, so the frilly frills and the awe of an anniversary had long gone for us: no flowers, no silk, and no pearls. We didn't subscribe to any of that nonsense anyway. We celebrated with a low-key dinner at a nearby Mediterranean restaurant. In our usual frugal fashion, we split a vegetarian plate and an order of roasted feta between the two of us.

My appetite was slowly coming back, but I wasn't too interested in feeling full. My mandatory "stool softener" prescription pills kept going in without anything coming out. I felt my body getting heavier and heavier with each meal, and without any indication that it would ever leave. I drank coffee. I ate fiber. I willed it to happen. The entire length of my intestine had dozed off without an alarm clock set. Finally, six days after surgery, my bowels officially moved. It was an event to celebrate. I felt so much lighter.

Several friends and family checked in on me via phone. Staff at Loyola called to see how I was feeling more than once over that week. Diane also called to see if I needed anything. My work pals sent flowers and chocolates. Mike and Tom took me to lunch spots nearby. Mat and I met our friend Ed Sadlowski at his favorite Greek restaurant in the city. While my mind was a hazy shade of acetaminophen, getting out of bed and moving helped my spirits and my energy level. Everyone was checking on me, and it was nice. But whenever the conversation shifted to how awesome I was for giving away my kidney, all I felt was what could be described as sorrow.

By the end of the week, my Facebook page had been filled with goodwill and admiration. Well-wishes and praise rained down on me in a most uncomfortable way. I appreciated the sentiment and the love, but it was hard to bear. I found myself tearing up more that week than I ever had. And for what?

It sometimes came out of nowhere. I'd be fine, then an incredible sorrow would creep in. That brick in your gut or that lump you feel in your throat once you've lost someone you love, that was what I was feeling. I didn't think I was grieving my surgery or my kidney. I was fully committed to that decision. But I was grieving something, and I didn't know what.

We checked out of the hotel, loaded up the car, and headed to Loyola for my check-up with Dr Milner. Everyone was happy to see how well I was getting around. Then, again, out of nowhere, I started to cry. Dr. Milner looked concerned. Mat looked concerned. Through my tears and my sniffles, I explained that I had no explanation. "I don't know why I'm crying." None of the people in the room had an explanation either. Dr. Milner asked if I regretted my decision to donate.

"No, not at all. But I don't know why this is happening," I said as I pointed to my face.

By the time I left the hospital, I had stopped crying and was my usual self. My labs were perfect, and my recovery was moving along. Everything about my donation had transpired as expected, aside from my peculiar stream of tears, with a mind of its own.

We ventured back to Northeast Indiana to prepare for the weekend nuptials of Mat's baby sister, Mollie. We were in charge of bringing the BBQ pulled pork, and the rolls. Yes, it's a funny thing for vegetarians to commit to, but we knew a guy, and the deal was sealed. It would be a chance to see a lot of the family at once and to get some of the awkwardness out of the way. Everyone in the family knew. I now had to answer for my actions.

I called Kay to let her and Dad know when we'd be home. Mat also called his dad. They all wanted to come by the house, if it was okay with me. By the time I got my slippers on, family started piling into the dining room, my parents and his, his brother, his sister, and the kids. Everyone wanted to check in on me. It felt very similar to the medical students in my hospital room. They were in the midst of something new and unknown.

When my nephew Jay saw me walk around the corner toward him, I sensed that the kids had no clear expectation about what condition I'd be in now that I was missing an organ. I don't think he expected me to be walking toward him, smiling to wrap him in a hug. Hell, I didn't fully know what to expect. The fact that I looked to be recovering so well, and that they could see me in good physical shape, helped to confirm to them that my surgery was less scary than anticipated.

Dad and Kay gave me a card with a magnet that had the same Dr. Seuss quote I read in the Loyola brochure: "To the world you may be one person, but to one person you may be the world." I put it on the fridge next to Rosie the Riveter. While he hated the idea of me having the surgery, I think Dad was proud that I did it, and maybe a bit astonished. But really, he should have predicted my approach from past childhood experiences. When he forbids me to do something, that's exactly what I'm most likely to do.

The strange thing about having something removed from your insides is that there's no way to verify that it's really missing. I'm not a conspiracy theorist or a sci-fi kind of person, but I did have this curiosity. Sure, there were taped-up incisions on my stomach, and I felt bloated and sore. Sure, I had been told my kidney was in Pennsylvania. But was it really? I peed the same after surgery as I had beforehand. Shouldn't I feel a difference? Perhaps this was a clear indication that I might have trust issues that needed to be resolved.

I went through an entire surgery and believed the result to be exactly what I signed up for. But without photographic evidence, without a video showing my kidney being pulled from my gut and put into a thermos, I had no way to confirm it. That lingered in the back of my mind for longer than it should have, I suspect.

My imaginings about what might have happened while I was

under the knife were wildly over-creative. That one piece of doubt could have been alleviated from my mind had I thought to ask for a picture to be taken of my kidney when they removed it. But I was new at this thing. If I were to do it all over again, I would have most definitely hired a videographer to confirm it all.

Chapter 12

# What's to Be Gained by Giving Something Away?

For the first two weeks after returning from Loyola, I chose to work from home to give myself an opportunity to regenerate. Dr. Milner said my body and my remaining kidney would need time to pick up the slack and feel normal again. Once a person is left with one kidney, it grows in size and ability to fulfill the additional responsibility,[44] but it takes time to do so. I felt groggy, so I relegated myself to laptop work, scheduling meetings and events for later in the month and drafting an editorial about the Indiana automotive industry.

I also took that time to attempt to connect with the people in my chain. Dr. Milner wanted me to be prepared to never hear from any of them, as is sometimes the case. Still, I wanted to give this first interaction with them my best shot. There wasn't a pressing need for me to have a serious relationship with any of them, to be invited over for cookouts, or to exchange cards during the holidays. I didn't donate my kidney with that expectation in mind. For me, I just wanted to know that they were okay and to tell them that I hoped they would have a good life.

Joanna from Loyola served as the middleperson in this exchange, since none of us knew each other or our names or addresses; she was the connector. This protocol was meant to protect any one of us who might have wanted to remain anonymous. She would receive my letter, then pass it along to the other transplant coordinator. That person would then pass it along to the person I wanted to receive it in the first place. Since each of us had our own transplant coordinator, they all had the same responsibility: connecting us if we wanted to be connected.

I mulled over what message I wanted to convey for a few days. My intention was to write the man in Pennsylvania who received my kidney and "the guy down the hall." Since both men were now intimately connected to me, well-wishes to them both made sense. Once I dropped it in the mail, Joanna would take it from there. No deadline or clock was running on how long this process took from the time I sent Joanna the letter to the time they received it. Maybe I would hear from them in a few weeks. Perhaps it would take a few months, or maybe that communication would never come.

My messages were charming. My jokes were funny. I asked questions. I offered my email address, mailing address, phone number, and Facebook handle. "It is my hope that you are getting your strength and your life back and that you will be able to drop me a line to let me know you are well," I wrote. No stone was left unturned to appeal to each of them to connect with me in some way. With Dr. Milner's voice in my head, I knew my letters might not be reciprocated, but I gave it one hell of an effort. My letters were sent, and then I moved on.

My temporary ten-pound weight restriction proved to be problematic during my recovery. Our old puppy, Solomon, had a tumor removed from his leg the week Mat and I were in Maywood. He and our other old-timer, Cirus, stayed at our Vet's office while we were gone. It was their first-ever sleepover away from home. When Mat picked them up, they both had a case of kennel cough and anxiety, and Sol could barely hobble.

To see our giant Siberian Husky wearing a plastic cone around his neck and a cast on his leg was so pitiful. He was uncomfortable and mad, and once he lay down, it was difficult to get back up. Just like me, Solomon needed to take it easy, but just like with me, it was hard to relax when you had to pee.

We were recovering together in the bedroom, me with my laptop in bed and Sol on the rug next to me. I could see his frustration every time he had to get up. His nails would slip on the hardwood floor as he tried to get a grip. Because he couldn't fit his cone-head through the doggie door, I had to get up to open the screen door for him. I should have predicted "Solomon-Gate" would happen while I was home alone, but I didn't.

Sol needed a lift, but no matter how hard he tried, he couldn't get his footing. He was weak and tired and needed someone to scoop him up off the floor and put him on his feet. He needed Mat. Even though he was a big, skinny ball of fur, he was still more than ten pounds. I couldn't lift Solomon by myself, but I still tried. Then, I cried. I didn't cry out of pain. I cried, again, for no reason at all.

I hovered over him but couldn't pull him up. Kneeling on the floor next to him, using just my arms, didn't work either. He was such a squirmer. He cried, then I cried. Even though he was at work thirty minutes away, I called Mat. He could tell I wasn't myself, having a meltdown over something so silly, but I had no control over such things during that time, and he sensed it. Mat was coming home.

For a while, I sat on the side of the bed, just staring at Sol in a daze. I couldn't help him get up to pee. What was the big deal, right? But in that moment, it was an iceberg of despair. Through the window, I could see Dad's driveway. He had come home from his route to eat lunch. I called to ask him to lift Sol, trying to sound as unfazed as I could so as not to worry him. By the time Mat got home, Sol was back on the floor with an empty bladder, and I was in bed staring at the TV. I wondered if my reaction to that stressful situation would become my new norm. Did I trade away my kidney for an extra dose of empathy?

The occasional sadness subsided after a few weeks at home, immersed in my work. I was myself again, focused and entirely with it, but that deep despair was concerning and unexplained. I could usually bury my feelings deep down into my soul where they couldn't see the light, but this time, I couldn't do that, and to have no control over my emotions was a new experience that I didn't want to revisit.

Calls and mail came in from friends, strangers, and everyone in between. We saw Mat's Uncle Steve at Mollie's wedding. He and Aunt Sue were the first to approach me and ask questions about my surgery. Uncle Steve was a double-lung transplant recipient, after having been diagnosed with pulmonary fibrosis years prior. Up until that point, I didn't really know much about Mat's Uncle Steve, other than he had new lungs, and they lived across town. We saw him at the annual Barth family Christmas party and at the annual Barth Family summer cookout. He was a union man. He was goofy and made the kids laugh at his jokes. Now, we had a connection.

I received a call from Tim Musser a few days later. Tim was very hard to forget, although I hadn't spoken to him in years. I used to take the same yoga class as Tim and his wife, Carol, at the YMCA, and Carol worked in the factory's office where Mat and I used to work. They had their own American Cancer Society Relay for Life team at the high school every year, and so did we. I didn't know much about Tim before that call, which would have explained his outreach to me.

It was Uncle Steve who told Tim about my surgery. Turns out, the two of them were dear friends and volunteered together, talking to the community about organ donation. This was all news to me. Uncle Steve, being a lung recipient, and Tim, being a kidney and pancreas recipient, made them a perfect match for palling around town. Considering they were both equally ornery and passionate about organ donation, they were quite the team.

Tim wanted to hear all about my surgery, why I did it, how I was feeling, and who had my kidney. He wanted to know it all. Then, he told me all about his health struggles, dialysis, and his transplant journey. Tim affirmed that even though he had to take 57 different pills every day to support his kidney and pancreas, he never felt better. While several family members and friends wanted to give him their kidney, Tim eventually received his gift of life from a 26-year-old woman who died from a brain aneurysm.

At the end of our conversation, Tim said something that will stay with me forever. "Most of us never got to meet our donors to thank them. But I can thank you. Thank you for what you've done." That was all it took for the tears to come. I did absolutely nothing for Tim, but he passed his gratitude for his donor on to me.

The following day, I received a call from Tim's friend Diana LeBrun. She was a union electrician with IBEW and was also a donor. She donated her kidney to a man named Jimmy, whom she heard about through her community channels, and her husband received a kidney from a living donor. Diana volunteered with Uncle Steve and Tim to talk about donation at events in our region. She also wanted to know all about my donation. Then, she, too, thanked me for becoming a donor.

The chain reaction of people wanting to talk to me about my donation continued for quite some time. Folks hearing about my kidney from that infamous small-town grapevine or our close-knit labor movement found ways to reach me. Dick Merin, the president of the UAW CAP Council, sent the loveliest card with an enrollment in the Ferdinand Benedictine Spiritual Association. From then on, the Sisters of St. Benedict would forever remember me in their daily prayers. Dave Kobiela, a steelworker out of the Dana plant, USW 903, sent a card that made me melt: "I just want to tell you how grateful I am to know you and to know that there are heroes like you in the world."

Goodwill gestures continued, and I kept getting choked up over them. Mat's sister, Sarah, was frequently spotted outside in our garden doing the weeding, so I didn't have that chore looming over my head or pushing on my poofy stomach. Dad spent countless hours in the yard mowing and whacking the weeds. Facebook was a perpetual haven for posts of admiration. It was all very, very intense.

The way it seemed, there were few people left in the world who didn't know about my kidney, and I supposed it was time for me to reach out to them, too. Through my calls and visits, I had gotten my donation blurb, essentially my elevator pitch, down well. I shared the kidney chain process, tidbits from the Katie Couric news segment, and the location of my kidney with anyone who asked. It was still emotionally challenging to receive affirming feedback after I talked, but I hoped that would go away the more I spoke. Much like stage fright, the more you do it, the less you feel stressed about it, right?

Through my work, I had built a relationship with the editor of our local newspaper, Dave Kurtz. *The Star* was the only paper in our area, although the Fort Wayne outlets covered our news and the broader region. I emailed Dave to let him know I had donated my kidney and was available to talk about it if he thought it was a worthwhile story to share with our community.

Dave assigned a reporter, Octavia Lehman, to speak with me right away. We met in town at the newspaper's office for the interview. I did my best to provide a clear explanation of what a kidney chain is, why donation is important, and what I wanted others to know about it. My nerves were on high alert as I tried not to come across as self-promoting. I wanted to appeal to people to help the cause without focusing on myself.

Octavia asked if I had any photos from my surgery to include in her story. Mat and I had taken a few pictures of me at my first, second, and third dinners. He also took photos of my incisions and of me lying half-baked in the hospital bed after surgery. All my choices were of me in a hospital gown, either in bed or with a plate of food in front of me. I chose the least gory picture of me lying in bed flashing my usual peace sign.

My sister came to visit from Ohio shortly after my interview with Octavia. As a family, we all went to Roger's Harvest House in Hamilton for breakfast. Unbeknownst to me, the neighborhood had already seen my face long before we parked in the lot that morning. It was an awkward experience to walk past *The Star* newspaper box in front of the restaurant and see myself on the front page. Right below the feature "Dekalb Jobless Rate Edges Higher" was my face and the title "Woman Donates Kidney to Stranger.[45]"

We bought a copy for seventy-five cents and took it inside. I cringed as I read it, anticipating a braggadocious tone that would ensure I'd never talk about my kidney again. Thankfully, it came across like the public service announcement I had hoped for. "Steury wants to increase people's chances of getting off the kidney waiting list. As of August 3rd, in Indiana, 1,255 people are waiting for kidney transplants... Nationally, 92,832 are waiting for kidneys."

The article flowed well, but key details needed work to emphasize better what I wanted to convey. The concept of a kidney chain and how mine evolved wasn't very clear. If I had never heard of one, I would still be confused after reading my own words in black and white. I wanted minds to be shifted by this newfound radical way to help people. A clearer explanation was needed. I knew I could do better. I knew I could do better for the cause.

Side note:

*In 2012, The Star reporters each shared their top five stories covered during the year. Octavia Lehman noted her article "Woman Donates Kidney to Stranger" as her second pick, "Story of the Year.[46]" Dad, who was a regular subscriber to the paper, begrudgingly broke the news to me. It was comical but completely understandable to me. In any contest, a story about classic cars, in a town devoted to its automotive heritage, would most definitely win over any news about my relocated organ.*

My critique of the article made me think about other ways I could get the message out without being the lone voice doing the talking. My strategic organizing brain kicked into gear. I reached out to a colleague from the Fort Wayne *Journal Gazette* and offered up an interview. They assigned a reporter to come to our house shortly thereafter. I saw that as my chance to introduce them to my pal Tim. He could help people relate to kidney recipients' perspectives and why donating was important. Plus, he was a certifiable goofball, so he would make for a good subject, I thought. Tim was more than happy to oblige.

Jacklyn Youhana spent about an hour talking with Mat, Tim, and me around the dining room table. I very carefully explained my kidney donation while Tim explained his kidney and pancreas transplant surgery. Mat played the role of the supportive partner, which he did effortlessly. We overloaded Jacklyn with information, and when she left, we hoped for the best.

A few days later, a photographer was sent to our house to take a photo of Mat and me. I was wearing my pajama pants, assuming this would be a waist-up passport photo. Instead, he had me sit cross-legged on the floor while Mat sat over me. My arm rested on his leg, and it felt very unnatural. I would never sit on the floor unless there were furry bellies to rub. It seemed strange, but I wasn't the professional in the room. I told myself, "Just sit there and smile, Rachel."

By the end of September, the greater metropolitan region of Northeast Indiana knew about my and Tim's innards. On the front page of the Living Section was this amber-hued photo of Mat and me.

The photographer had captured the warmth of the copper paint on the wall, the woodwork, and the colors in my shirt like a pure artist. All that hullabaloo on the floor with the weird arm setup happened because he was setting the perfect scene.

"Kidney's Gone, Heart is Intact. Auburn Woman Becomes Good Samaritan Donor" was the title Jacklyn chose.[47] She not only interviewed me, Mat, and Tim, but also reached out to the National Kidney Registry and interviewed Garet Hil. Her article was thorough as hell, with statistics and processes, peppered with feel-good quotes from all of us. She even reviewed the Katie Couric segment so she could explain how Max Zapata's donation chain worked.

Jacklyn wrote a very detailed article about my donation that didn't center me. It again affirmed that my story could be told in a way that focused on the need, without too much emphasis on me. She gave me the confidence to keep talking without the fear of sounding pretentious.

A week later, Mat came home from work and, with a smile, gave me a large envelope. Inside was "The Herald," a newspaper from Dubois County, Indiana. Dubois was so far south that it was almost in Kentucky. A colleague of Mat's read our story in his local newspaper and mailed it to him. "Indiana Woman Donates Kidney to Stranger" was the title.[48] It was half of the text from the *Journal Gazette* article, still attributed to Jaclyn, of course. I didn't realize at the time that a local article published in one newspaper could also be published in multiple others. I thought that only happened with articles from the Associated Press. After I read that article, I was curious where else our story might have landed. That's when I took a breath and googled myself.

The hits that popped up in my search made my heart race. It was no longer a Northeast Indiana story, nor was it relegated to the confines of a black and white newspaper. It was out there for the world to read. Blogs, medical journals, faraway newspapers; my kidney was news. My initial feeling of being overwhelmed by the notoriety eventually gave way to a comfortable sigh. People who may not have known beforehand now know that someone ordinary like me gave away a kidney in a way that had the potential to catch on. There I was, being the vessel for the cargo. There I was.

Our nieces and nephews took an interest in the local buzz around town. Aunt Rae had made the front page of the paper, and it wasn't the police blotter. A couple of the kids took my article to school for show-and-tell. I wish I could've been a fly on the wall to hear them explain this complicated system from their perspective.

As time went on, my work life and kidney life began to intersect in a way I hadn't anticipated. Whenever I did a presentation about manufacturing for a group who knew me personally or read an article about me, they would out me during introductions. It was peculiar at first to have that deed on everyone's mind as I spoke about the manufacturing multiplier effect and Midwest shipments of feedstock across the globe. I was sure it distracted from the impressive trade statistics and policy ideas I really wanted them to absorb instead.

Oftentimes, the last question during a presentation would be an ask for me to share my story with them. I became pretty good at the very condensed version of my kidney donation: my birthday, Katie Couric, my kidney is in Pennsylvania, the need is great, and anyone can sign up to be a potential donor. This is when standing ovations began.

I rarely received a standing ovation for my manufacturing presentations, for my glossy handouts, or for my funny jokes about being the *President of the Charts and Graphs Fan Club*. Yet there I was with rooms full of folks on their feet, smiling up at me. Going from being painfully reserved when talking about myself to having people of all political stripes, ages, and classes feel moved by the thing I did felt uncomfortable and inspiring at the same time. It made me feel like my voice mattered more than I gave it credit for. Maybe they could envision themselves telling a similar story.

What impacted me the most about sharing my story within the labor movement and the various social groups in our region was meeting people who were intimately connected to this new world I had entered. They'd come up after my presentations to thank me for my work and for my donation. Then, they would share their own stories with me. There was always one person who knew a recipient, was a recipient themselves, or had a deceased donor, like my Uncle

Ed, in their lives. Some were still waiting for the call that an organ was available for them, waiting on the list that never got shorter.

Before my surgery, the only recipient I knew was Uncle Steve, and the only donor I knew was Uncle Ed. I was the lone kidney donor in my life, but that began to change with every elevator pitch I gave. People in this organ donation community started popping out of the woodwork, and it made my world feel much bigger.

I, however, still felt very isolated in my experience as a donor. Aside from Diane from NKR, Diana, Tim's friend, and Barb from Loyola, I knew no one like me. Sure, I had read newspaper articles about other donors, and Max Zapata was in my mind, but a real-life person standing in front of me with a similar experience was lacking in my life. I was indeed a unicorn. I didn't know anyone like me, and I wanted to.

Months after my face was plastered on the front page, I stopped in our vet's office to get heartworm medication for the dogs. When the staff noticed me walk in, a silence came over the place, and I wasn't sure what I was walking into. Did a dog die today? Are we mourning a loss here?

Roxy, the technician we had come to love, thanked me for being a donor. She said one of the other techs in the office was on dialysis and needed a kidney transplant. He was sick, and they hoped to find someone to donate to him. She then shared that her husband and his twin brother were both in need of kidney transplants. They had polycystic kidney disease, a genetic disease, and were very sick. She and the family were searching for donors.

My heart ached for them, and at the same time, I felt a bit of guilt. Three people connected to our vet's office needed a kidney, and mine was now hundreds of miles away. In my excitement and determination to start a kidney chain, I never thought to ask around town, "Hey, do you know someone who needs my kidney?"

For a myriad of reasons, folks don't talk about their failing health. To make a plea to strangers in everyday conversation was an unnatural thing to do. Much like I had to convince myself to talk about my donation, those on the other end of this exchange also had to be convinced to be vulnerable and to ask for help publicly.

If my Grana had kept her stories to herself, if she had allowed my Uncle Ed's death and his donation to remain in the silent sanctuary of her heart, I might still have two kidneys. By allowing herself to be vulnerable enough to talk about such a traumatic loss, she gave new life to others. By allowing myself to be the voice for the message, the vessel carrying the cargo, I hoped to enable others to have hope and inspiration for what might come.

# Chapter 13

# **My Family Tree Adds a Branch**

It was mid-September when I received mail from Loyola. The smaller envelope inside the bigger envelope was unsealed and just had my first name on it. Inside was a letter addressed, *To My Donor*. It felt very much like an exchange made within a prison system. If you write a letter to an inmate or an inmate writes one to you, the jailers are sometimes required to read the letters first to ensure there is no funny business taking place, no elaborate schemes to escape, and no hits ordered on anyone on the outside.

"My name is Harry, and I live in Illinois," the letter began. He shared details about his life, his family, and his health. He worked for an airline and had a big, close-knit family. He loved to sing and bowl and had just recently been baptized. Harry wrote about how long he had been in need of a kidney. Finally, he was feeling well and able to get back to living.

"I thank you so much, and my family is very grateful."

Harry provided his mailing address in the event his donor wanted to reach out to him. I had a feeling Harry wrote more than one letter, just like I did. Perhaps both donors in our chain received mail from him that day. His letter was written to me without him knowing who any of us were at the time, just like I wrote mine.

Finally, the "guy down the hall" had a name. A few days after that, Harry also had a phone number, a Facebook page, an email address, and a face. That was when Harry finally received my letter with all my contact information and began his own mission of securing our connection. My first text from Harry included pictures of him sitting on a couch surrounded by his wife, Pat, and his grandchildren. He followed up the text with an email containing more photos of him and his kids. Next, I received his Facebook friend request, and then finally, Harry called.

I knew I loved Harry the moment I heard his voice. He had no idea how much it meant for me to know that he was doing okay. Harry was a religious person, and he thanked his God for me, and his congregation did the same. I think it's correct to assume that Harry's faith played a tremendous role in his valiant effort to reach out to me.

It was hard for me to stay composed on the call with Harry. To have someone directly involved in our kidney chain thank me for my role in it was very real and raw. Hearing Harry's voice and knowing he was physically, emotionally, and spiritually impacted by this decision made my heart nearly burst. And to think, some folks never get to know who anyone is in their chain, but as Dr. Milner explained, we had to be okay with that.

Harry and I declared that we'd stay in touch, and we planned to meet in person the next time I was working in the Chicago area. He asked me about the other people in our chain, but the only thing I had to share was that my kidney went to a man in Pennsylvania. Harry told me he had written his donor, too, but had not heard from her. All he knew was that his donor was a woman.

Two weeks later, I received mail from Pennsylvania. This time, there was no middleman and no coordination on anyone's part. My Pennsylvania connection used the contact information from my letter to write directly to me. Indeed, all that charm and humor I poured into my letters had paid off, just as I hoped.

My recipient was unable to write me because he was "not much of a writer," but his wife wasted no time taking on the task. "I happen to be married to the man you so generously donated your kidney to," the letter explained. She went on to tell me about their family and her husband's health. I also learned about the second donor, the woman who gifted Harry his new kidney so that her uncle could receive mine.

My recipient's wife shared their occupations and that he was already back at work. Then she ended her letter with well wishes. "Again, we thank you from the bottom of our hearts for what you have done and pray that you may always keep your good health."

Her words were all I needed from this transaction. My kidney allowed someone to get back to living, and he was okay. I understood, from my discussion with Dr. Milner, that it could feel impossible for a recipient to write a thank-you note to their donor. When there weren't words to adequately describe what someone has done for you, "Thank You" doesn't seem like enough. For me, it was enough.

By the time that letter arrived, *The Star* and *Journal Gazette* articles had already been published. I sent a follow-up letter to Pennsylvania and enclosed the *Journal Gazette* article. I asked a few questions about their work in case they wanted to respond or stay in touch, as Harry did. As an organizer, I was always compelled to bring people together. If I could do that with the people in my chain, that would be phenomenal.

Two months passed before I accepted that my outreach efforts would not be reciprocated. My recipient didn't anticipate an extended family out of this deal any more than I did. I knew the odds were slim for me to even hear from him, much less for us to become inseparable friends forever. Alas, there would be no annual potluck at the neighborhood park, no Secret Santa gift exchanges at the Eagles, no meeting with all of us joining together on the couch in Max Zapata's house for a big family photo op.

My recipient simply wanted a kidney. And considering his family member donated her kidney on his behalf, he most assuredly saw her as the donor in his life. While I gave him the kidney, she gave him the golden ticket to get it. Both of us were his donor. I could appreciate him feeling reserved about putting himself out there. Believe me, I understood that feeling.

For this reason, I have left my recipient and his family's names out of this memoir to respect their privacy. If they ever want to reconnect with me, I would absolutely welcome it. My only hope out of this exchange was to hear from both recipients to know they were okay. Then I could happily move on, knowing that they were.

At the end of October, Mat and I made the trip to Chicago to meet Harry and his wife, Pat, at their house. I had zero expectations for how our first encounter would go, aside from hoping to stay fully composed. We were meeting perfect strangers, yet we had a connection that was more personal than anyone else we technically didn't know.

I knocked on the front door and waited barely a second for it to open. Staring back at me was a bright-eyed man with a glowing smile. If Harry or I said anything when we first laid eyes on each other, I don't recall. We hugged for what felt like an hour as Pat stepped around the corner to offer her own hug. They instantly felt like family.

We spent half of the day talking and eating at the Panera Bread near their house. During our marathon lunch, we got to know them and their family, and they got to know ours. Had it not been for this kidney chain, the likelihood that we would have ever crossed paths was slim to none. To me, that would have been an unfortunate loss. To never know Harry and Pat and how terrific they are would have been a shame. This leads me to wonder, how many of those people sitting in the nearby booths at that Panera Bread were brought together simply because of the Broccoli Cheddar Soup? What magical conversations were taking place, not because of the Mediterranean Veggie Sandwich, but in spite of it?

Mat and I were so different from Harry and Pat in our life experiences, our spirituality, and our cultural influences, yet there we were absorbed in conversation about my and Pat's careers, Mat's Amish bloodline, and Harry's childhood path from the Philippines. I deeply appreciated having two such genuine and caring people officially in our lives, and their family unit, a solid, fully connected family tree with nary a broken or tattered limb, was something to be admired. They were the family members I never knew were missing.

Harry and I planned to stay in touch, and we absolutely have. With every check-up appointment and blood test, Harry has called me with an update on his health. I called him when I had my check-ups, too. We have been personally invested in each other's well-being, celebrating every creatinine check together.

Four months had passed since my donation, and Mat and I were running out of days in 2012 to choose the race we would run. We waited until the last possible moment before we finally settled on

Thanksgiving Day to honor our New Year's resolution. The first race of our lives would be The Galloping Gobbler. Thousands of people from Northeast Indiana flocked, or galloped, to participate in this race every year before strapping on the feedbag for the long day of overconsumption. We decided 2012 was a good time to join them.

I was nervous about the event for several reasons. We had to get up early to make the drive to Fort Wayne, and my internal alarm clock hated mornings. Plus, my love of coffee had to wait until after the race because I'd have to pee when I was supposed to be running. Most importantly, I didn't want to slow Mat down.

He was taller than me and had always been more active, even before we met. My dad's idea of me playing sports consisted of a Saturday morning bowling league. Mat wasn't in many organized sports either, but his mode of transportation and enjoyment was often inline skates and skateboards. While we both actively went to the gym, kickboxing, and yoga classes as adults, he was still taller than me by about half a foot. Did I mention he was taller than me?

My lack of a kidney was of no concern in this equation. I was feeling fine, though Dad thought the idea of running anytime, much less so soon after surgery, was unwise. He felt protective about a lot of things all my life, but if he couldn't stop me from giving away a kidney, he wasn't changing my mind about a four-mile race. If I stayed focused on the turtle analogy, slow and steady would win the race for me. I wasn't vying to technically win any race; I simply wanted to finish it. That was what winning meant to me. To finish was to win.

Mat and I started the race together as planned. The noises and the aggression of the runners around me made me feel like I had to run faster and faster, even though I was barely at a jog to begin with. I lost steam quickly. As I began to move slower and slower, so did Mat. He could have lapped me three times, you know, because he was taller than me, but he didn't. Even when I told him to go ahead of me, he wasn't leaving my side.

We finished the Galloping Gobbler together, right in the middle of the pack of three thousand gallopers. While that was a New Year's resolution to check off the list, it was also an indicator of what Mat and

I determined to be important components of our lives. We continued to challenge each other to be better versions of ourselves. We were on this adventure together, no matter where the road or the finish line would lead us.


Joanna, from Loyola, sent me an email early in 2013 about the National Kidney Registry's gala. She said they put on the event every year, and I was invited as a 2012 NKR donor. It would be at the Waldorf Astoria in New York City, and if I were interested, she could get us tickets.

It sounded very exciting, but like a good researcher, I needed more information. What was the location? How much did it cost? Could Harry and Pat come with us? It sounded like something I had to wrap my mind around, to prepare for. Joanna did her best to explain what I could expect. From the sound of it, this was a black-tie event, and I would be surrounded by elegance. It was a celebration of the donors and the transplant teams from the previous year and all that the NKR had accomplished. NKR also presented an award to each donor, and there would be a lot of handshaking and fancy food-eating.

Attending the gala was free, but the other costs, like getting there and staying there, were not. NKR had a block of rooms reserved at the Waldorf Astoria for the low, low price of $395 a night. Flights in and out of the city were not cheap. My frugal mind wrestled with the thought of spending so much money for a one-night event while at the same time wanting to jump right into this new club I had inadvertently joined.

Mat would not let me pass up the opportunity to attend, no matter how expensive it was. We confirmed with Joanne, and we were formally invited. We planned to spend the extended weekend in the city to explore and enjoy. I scoured the web for better hotel rates at places near the Waldorf Astoria to no avail. Finally, I settled on reserving one $395 night there and then cashing in all my accumulated hotel points from my work trips for two nights at a hotel farther away. We bought a few Groupons for cheap meals around the city. We swallowed hard as we dropped $1,000 on flights, but it was confirmed that we were headed to the Gala.

I thought a lot about those Gala expenses. How many donors could afford to spend over $1,500 to eat dinner in New York City? In my reality, disposable income like this wasn't commonplace. A week-long vacation for an entire family wouldn't cost $1500, but there we were spending it for three nights in the city. The term "valuable consideration" mentioned in my pre-donation paperwork ran through my mind. This seemed like one of those fuzzy scenarios that could be interpreted as a violation of the law, if not handled appropriately. Of course, donors had to pay their own way to an event like this. If donors received an all-expenses-paid trip to New York City to celebrate their donation of a kidney, that could be considered payment.

Who would be attending the Gala was a wonder to me, too. I knew there'd be other donors, which I was excited about. To be in a roomful of people like me and not feel like the unicorn was something I could only imagine. But if we spent $1,500 to make the trip, others would have to as well, unless they were all locals. Did all donors within NKR have this kind of means? Would I *really* be in a room full of people like me?

During our flight into the city, I wrote up my notes. If awards were to be given out, I would have to have a clever speech in exchange. While I knew I probably could not get through any lengthy presentation without choking up, I had to be prepared to say something: Veggie Stix, Dr. Milner, the guy down the hall. I was as ready as I was going to be.

Walking through the doors of the Waldorf Astoria felt like an out-of-body experience. In normal times, the likes of me would never be invited into a place like that, but there I was, checking in. When we got to our room, it was clear that the more money you pay for a hotel room, the fewer amenities they provide; no coffee maker, no fridge, no internet. This was definitely not the LaQuinta Inn. It must be some reverse psychology game played by the elite. Less is more, so just appreciate the thread count.

Mat and I cleaned up pretty well. He wore the tie I got him from the Senate gift shop and that American-made dress shirt from the Curiosity Shop. I wore a dress that was two sizes too big because it was $5 at Goodwill, and I liked it. It complemented Grana's pearls around my neck. My not-so-fancy Georgia-made Okabashi's played a starring role as the only black dress shoes I had. No one would be looking down at my feet anyway.

We entered the banquet room and were instantly dazzled. Everything was sparkly, from the chandeliers to the table settings. There was assigned seating, and we joined a collection of smiling people around an overly accessorized table. The room felt small but was overflowing with charming people and shiny salad forks.

It was humbling to sit in a room full of donors. I couldn't distinguish the surgeons from the donors, so we talked to the people at our table over dinner and found donors in our midst. That is where we met Ray Mueller, a non-directed donor from New Jersey, and Lloyd Withers, a non-directed donor from New York. Both were soft-spoken and friendly, and we hit it off. There were other people like us all over that banquet hall, but I stayed in my seat and got to know my tablemates.

In my occupation, I would have worked that room like nobody's business to meet as many people as possible and find as many donors as possible. But I was overwhelmed by the scene, so I stayed inside myself that night. It was an emotional overload to finally be with people like me. I wanted to know all of them. I also wanted just to breathe and take it all in. Plus, I still had a speech to give. I had to reserve my strength for the public speaking we were all about to do.

As the meal wrapped up, the founder of NKR, Garet Hil, appeared on the stage. He looked just as glamorous in real life as he did with Katie Couric in 2010: sharp suit, magazine smile. He's one of those people who don't age. Perhaps he's made a deal with the Devil, or Saint Peter, or both.

A series of speeches from medical personnel ensued. Awards were presented to surgeons and transplant teams. Accolades were given. Sitting on the table to the side of the stage was a collection of awards that looked like skyscrapers. Tall, rectangular pieces of metal with red glass running up the sides of them. They were to be presented to the donors. One of them was coming home with us.

Whatever Garet said at that point was a blur. I remember being teary-eyed as admiration was piled upon the donors in the room, with

Mat staring lovingly back at me. I took my notes with me as Garet called each of our names, one by one, to present the award and to take the stage together. When the last of us were on the stage, the room stood in ovation. It was painful. I cried, staring out into the audience at Mat, who was perpetually smiling back at me. I was clutching my notes, still very ready to thank the NKR for championing this cool new way to help people.

When the ovation finally ended, the hand gesture from the usher next to the stage signaled that it was time to go back to our tables. I turned to look at the microphone; no one was standing in front of it. My gut reaction was to grab the mic and start talking, but that may have gotten us kicked out of my new club, or certainly would have gotten my award revoked. I walked off the stage and sat down, unsettled.

That was the first awards ceremony I had ever attended in which the award recipients remained silent. There would be no "thanking of the academy" or drawn-out speeches where the orchestra would play anyone off the stage for talking too long. Maybe NKR assumed donors wouldn't want to talk. Maybe past galas proved that to be true. The fact that none of us spoke was a relief to me, but also made me question why. It would be years before I learned just how many non-directed donors were natural-born, hard-core introverts. It wasn't just me. Talking about ourselves could be downright excruciating.

As the evening wound down, we were all invited to take the leftover wine from the tables with us to our rooms. On our way out of the banquet hall with our stash, we came across Garet Hil in the hall. I felt like that might be my only opportunity to impart words on the guy, so I did.

I introduced myself and Mat to him and thanked him for his work. Then, like a groupie, I asked for a picture. He obliged, maintaining that magazine smile the whole way through. Another donor and her husband had the same idea in mind, so we helped each other take photos with the person who helped us give away our kidneys. The man, who, for the love of his own daughter, helped tons of people live by sharing his smarts and their story with the masses.

When we got back home, I dug out the award, which was wrapped snuggly in my pajama pants in our checked bag. What was once a towering skyscraper just the day before had become a double-wide trailer. The award had broken in two pieces during transit. Having welders in our crew makes a big difference in situations like this. You know, when your kidney skyscraper breaks in half, who're you gonna call? Thanks to our pal Shippy, who made it as good as new.

If I were a believer in signs, which I often am, I might have concluded that the break was supposed to happen. A tower-turned-double-wide might be just the message we need to hear sometimes. An award tells the tale that we have somehow achieved something higher than those without one. They are flamboyant. They are showboat-y. They recognize us for our outstanding X, Y, and Z. They can make us cocky. They can also set us apart and make our experiences seem unreachable.

People needed to see that living donors were just like them if we were going to create a space for more people to choose to become one. I am a normal, everyday kind of person who happened to do this thing that could someday catch on to be very common. The day there are more people with one kidney than two may become a reality if we captivate the hearts and minds of those ready to make it so. If we are so damned relatable that people can see themselves in us, they just may.

I understand an award like that could be an excellent conversation starter at the next holiday gathering or Lions Club meeting hosted in one's living room, but I had to disconnect the deed from the praise. My feelings about its real message remain today. It is a constant reminder to always stay humble in our deeds and, for crying out loud, don't get cocky because of the inventory on the mantle.

Chapter 14

# The Evolution of My Origin Story

Tim Musser reentered my life after my donation, and he did so in a significant way. He continued to pour his admiration for his own donor onto me with phone calls on a regular basis, and I welcomed it. We'd often have breakfast at his favorite local spot, the Northway Inn, and shoot the breeze. We were just two union people with loads of stories to share, his time in the shop as an autoworker, and mine as a steelworker. He had a big heart, and I was glad to be sharing this world with him.

Tim invited me to attend a new volunteer orientation at IOPO, where he and Uncle Steve did their outreach. He referred to it by its acronym as if it were a word: eye-OH-poe. Once he explained to me what that meant, I dug deep into the back of my mind to find the reference. The Indiana Organ Procurement Organization, or IOPO for short, was new to me but still oh-so-familiar.

My family had a brief history with them. This was the same group that existed back in 1990 when Uncle Ed died. IOPO rang a bell for me because it was the organization that sent my Grana her coveted letter —the one that informed her of how many lives Uncle Ed saved, the one she kept in every drawer in the house.

At the time, I was still traveling often for work and didn't have the bandwidth to commit to anything else. I was already talking with people about kidney donation during intermissions from my work presentations. Still, I found myself curious enough to attend the orientation to see what it was all about. Tim lit up when he talked about the outreach he and Uncle Steve were doing with IOPO. Maybe I would, too.

Because of his health conditions, Tim had been declared legally blind. To navigate the roads around our small town, he wore very sophisticated headgear that amplified his surroundings enough to drive. They reminded me of the military night vision contraptions you see in the movies. He drove very well with those things, but tackling Interstate 69 to get to the IOPO office in Fort Wayne? Thankfully, he left the driving to me.

IOPO was tucked into a building in the business district near Jefferson Point, set off the road with a lone sign indicating what was inside. The meeting was scheduled to be just a few hours long, and because of Tim, everyone knew who I was before I walked through the door. As we entered the office, Tim called out to people he walked past, introducing me by name and by deed. "This is my friend Rachel, and she just did something really special."

I met the regional volunteer coordinators, Marti Cooper and Kelli Luckett. They were the staff members who arranged all the volunteer assignments and outreach for volunteers like Tim and Uncle Steve. They also did the training and kept the program as publicly visible as possible. We walked into the conference room to meet the rest of the folks participating that day. I didn't know any of them, but Tim made sure to remedy that in a matter of minutes.

The orientation began with a tour and an explanation of what IOPO was. I was intrigued. As Indiana's designated organ procurement organization, IOPO did the crucial work of talking with families when their loved ones died. They consoled people who were grieving while at the same time allowing them the opportunity to find solace through organ donation. IOPO not only did the tough work of communicating appropriately with donor families, but also facilitated connections between donated organs and patients in need on the waitlist. To top it off, IOPO also employed specialists in the recovery of organs for transport to their designated recipients.

The mission of the IOPO volunteer program was to end the waitlist. That meant volunteers would encourage as many people as possible to become registered eye, organ, and tissue donors. Since most people made that decision at the DMV when they first got or renewed their driver's licenses, IOPO volunteers reached a small percentage of the population: those who were holding out on making the decision or teenagers who would soon have their first DMV experience.

I was unaware of all that IOPO did in the lifesaving arena, and I certainly never would have guessed it had a volunteer component. As a young person, seeing Grana's prized letter, I had little reason to know more about the group than that it was an informant, churning out letters to donor families when the need arose. To be such an impactful part of the state's history and to connect donors with recipients as the designated group for the area was impressive. I soon learned every state had at least one organization like this.

Wrapped around a large conference table, I met people who were connected to donation in very different ways. Folks like Tim and Uncle Steve, who were celebrating their new lease on life, were there. They were hopeful, proud, and ready to tell the world about their new heart, lungs, or kidney. Also, at the table were people like my Grana, who were mourning the loss of a family member who became a donor in the end. There were also caregivers at the table. Nursing a spouse or child back to health from a lifetime of illness toward an eventual transplant is challenging work. They had a unique perspective on how important donation was to a family unit. Then, there was me.

As each person introduced themselves and explained what brought them to the meeting, I could feel the collective pain in the room. I could also feel the joy. Those who were celebrating their new organs were also mourning the life that was lost for them to be able to live on. Those who were mourning the loss of their child or sibling were also celebrating the lives that were saved because of their gift. I was overwhelmed, and so were my tear ducts.

It was an unconventional space where people grieved and rejoiced at the same time. By talking about their loved one who died or their donors who gave them life, bonds were formed. It was a literal support group for life and death. As volunteers, they were learning how to take all that emotion and honor their loved ones by doing the work. By sharing tidbits of their stories and registering people in our region to become donors, they were giving themselves permission to heal and move forward. They were allowing joy to outwit their grief.

I wondered how Grana would have felt around a table like that when Uncle Ed's death was still raw. Would she have embraced the idea of bonding with recipients as a way to honor her son? By the time I learned of IOPO and was in that room full of volunteers, Grana was not very active in the world. Broken bones and the ailments of age relegated her to her favorite chair, where she watched The Price Is Right most days. She was present, but her mind had begun to wander.

Sitting at the meeting alongside so many people touched by donation in one way or another, I felt very much at home while also feeling like an outsider. I was the lone donor in the room again. I took that as an opportunity to build upon. Since there weren't too many people like me to begin with, perhaps I would be the person to bring them into the fold. Perhaps, through this volunteer gig, I could start by being the change I wanted to see.

In my mind, all the people we could approach about registering to become deceased donors in the future were potential living donors in the present. A story like mine, in this environment, could compel people to donate an organ without waiting for death to give them that opportunity. How I would arrive at that point in a discussion with others had to be thoughtful and kind, and my story couldn't lead anyone to think that living donation was my only ask. My ask would be multi-fold.

"Consider registering to be an organ donor in whatever way you choose, through deceased donation once you've passed away, or through living donation, to give a part of yourself to someone who needs you now. Both are honorable, and either one will do."


A few months had passed from that initial meeting, and Marti invited me to participate in a storytelling class that IOPO was organizing for some of their volunteers. Because I did a lot of public speaking in my work, she thought it would be a good class for me to learn tips for telling donation stories in my volunteer capacity. Not all IOPO volunteers were comfortable with standing up in front of groups, but she knew this had become part of my profession. And perhaps she also knew I needed to be smoked out of my foxhole. I needed to be smoked out of my very surface-level-elevator-speech foxhole.

Brianna Doby flew in from Colorado to put on the workshop. She did this for a living for many organ procurement organizations across the country through her company, "Positive Rhetoric." I had never heard of her or her company, but I had been a lifelong learner and would be the first to confess that I still have not learned it all.

Ahead of the in-person meeting, Brianna asked attendees to write a five-minute speech. She wanted us to write the speech as if speaking to a group about registering to become donors, with our own personal tidbits about donation included, so that folks had a human connection to why it was so important. Then, we were to email our drafts to her before our workshop so she could review them and be prepared to offer feedback when we were all together.

A five-minute speech is about 750 words, one chunky full page. I wasn't used to writing legitimate speeches. In my work, I would create an outline of topics I wanted to cover and then speak from those notes. It was a way to force myself to know what I was talking about without having the cheat sheet in front of me. My process made me engage with the eyes in the room, not the words on the paper. Writing a speech felt clunky to me, but I wasn't one to not turn in my homework assignments either.

My speech began in my comfort zone, with the facts and the numbers: 3.4 million Hoosiers were registered donors, a single donor could save eight lives, 18 people died each day waiting for an organ, and so on. It was peppered with humor about "having a heart" and joining the cool kids who register to become donors. It began as a speech that anyone could tell, regardless of their personal connection.

While my typical elevator speech usually stopped short of detailing my donation decision, this iteration was the first time I incorporated Uncle Ed and Grana into my public testimony. They had always been a part of my origin story, but typing the words, much less saying them, proved to be most difficult for me. Still, I typed them. For this speech, the references to Uncle Ed and Grana were exactly seventy-five words. Just three whole sentences of my one-page speech were about them. That was the extent of what I thought I could project out into the universe while still maintaining my composure.

With my focus being on the need and the numbers, there just wasn't room for any more of my personal details. There were facts to present, and dammit, that was gonna move people. My own kidney donation encompassed six sentences, with Katie Couric receiving the starring role. I ended the speech with my call to "have a heart" and register to become a donor.

I emailed my speech to Brianna and predicted what our future encounter would look like. I'd eventually have to say the thing out loud in front of a roomful of people. In doing so, she'd tell me how to make it better. I would also ugly-cry and constrict inside of my skin. At the end of the workshop, I'd have a stress headache and leave the room feeling like I needed a beer. Wouldn't you know, that's exactly what happened.

"Have you ever heard the term 'bury the lead?' Because that's what you just did, Rachel."

She said it in the nicest possible way, as the other volunteers shook their heads in agreement. The focus of my story wasn't me; it was the need. Brianna offered a few suggestions for bringing my speech to life. I could hold up a section of a chain to symbolize a kidney chain. Instead of talking about having the heart on my driver's license, I could flash my own driver's license for people to see what I was talking about.

When she made the connection between my Uncle Ed and my recipient in Pennsylvania, I felt like I was in therapy, discovering a breakthrough I never knew I needed. Brianna suggested I take a photo of Uncle Ed with me for my speeches and, if I had one, a photo of my recipient, and then set the two photos next to each other. Because while Uncle Ed saved the lives of five people in 1990, he also saved the life of my recipient in Pennsylvania, twenty-two years after his death.

"They have never met, but one saved the other's life," Brianna explained.

She went on for what seemed like days about all the ways I could tell my story, many of which were too personal for me to entertain. My ability to stay composed and tell the story conflicted with the way the story needed to be told. This is what happens when you're surrounded by people who don't show their feelings or talk about the hard stuff. Aside from my Grana, no one spoke about their trauma or their accomplishments, and I didn't either.

At the end of her critique, Brianna went in for the kill, unloading buckets of admiration upon me in my weakest of moments. That's when the ugly crier in me was front and center.

"You have a lovely way of interacting with people. I know you wanna get up there and be like, 'I'm no big deal,' but you're a big frickin deal! Oh my God, Rachel, you just woke up one day and saved somebody's life. If I can raise my children to be the kind of person that you are, that's my dream."

By that time, I wasn't the only one in tears. The whole room had joined me. Brianna turned to Marti and suggested that me doing speeches alongside someone else would be a good compromise. I wasn't going to talk myself up, so someone else needed to do that for me.

"Do your talks with somebody who can show you off because I know you can't do that yourself. You're much too humble."

It's a good thing I had Tim.

What I learned in that workshop led me to reflect on the whys and hows of my own life. Why are the words so hard to say? How did I become the one to do this thing so few consider doing? The other storytellers in the room that day spoke to me in a very tangible way. My new community at IOPO was made up of people just like me, long before I donated my kidney.

Many of the other storytellers were family members of loved ones who died unexpectedly or prematurely through tragic accidents or suicide. They were donor moms, sisters, and grandfathers who held onto the grief of death but turned it into positive advocacy. Up until that point, I had hoarded more than my fair share of that kind of sorrow, too, but I still wasn't fully equipped to turn it into an all-out campaign.

My storytelling abilities were junk because the feelings and the words I needed to convey the message confidently had been buried for decades. Being able to talk about death freely wasn't a thing anyone in my family was accustomed to, other than my Grana. As a kid, she talked at me more than she talked with me. On many of our road trips across the Midwest, she'd glance back at me through the rear-view mirror to see if I was paying attention. I'd have my head down as if I didn't care and wasn't listening, but I did care, and I was most definitely listening. As a young person, it was just too painful to be present in those conversations.

For as long as I have been alive, my family has been held together by a bond of trauma. Shared experiences of grief and sorrow, peppered with a will to overcome, solidified our coalition and designated Grana our top executive. We would walk this earth proudly, but with baggage and burden impossible to shake. To appear completely unfazed by the happenings of the past was something I became good at because I tucked away my feelings and never spent any time exploring them. At the same time, that learned defense mechanism was boring a hole into my soul.

When Uncle Ed died, he was Grana's second child to die by suicide, using a gun. While Uncle Ed made it just past his 27th birthday, my mother, Joy, lived to the ripe old age of 21. Grana's birthday was the day my mother picked up the gun. Her own mother's birthday. Mental illness is hard to escape, no matter how hard you try.

My mother left behind my dad, my sister, and me in what was an obvious case of post-partum depression, by all accounts. Even the medical examiner listed that as her cause of death. Forty years ago, few people knew how to treat it or what it could compel people to do to themselves or others. Grana said all the signs were there that she needed help, but no one knew how to help. Only in the past few decades has post-partum depression been acknowledged for its intensity and repercussions.

Depression in women after childbirth is more common than many realize, but the extent to which self-harm or suicidal thoughts enter the mind varies. Physical or sexual abuse as a child or adult, sleep deprivation, or anxiety-related disorders are some of the underlying issues that contribute to the intensity of these feelings.[49] Sleep deprivation is an absolute consequence of being a new parent, unless you have a live-in nanny on staff. So is anxiety, but in the 1970s, who would have thought to connect those dots and conjure up a way to resolve it?

I remember the confidence Uncle Ed had when I was a kid. I never remembered him being down or depressed, but still, he was. He presented to the world an unfazed version of himself, all the while fighting his own internal war. My uncle was pronounced dead on the very same day my beautiful cousin, Sam, was born. She would never know her father, just as I would never know my mother.

Grana was the only one to talk about them freely. She was the portal to the pain, but she kept on talking because that was the only way any of us were going to know who her kids were. Plus, I think she needed to keep them alive in her own mind. It was her way to grieve and to ensure we knew what kind of people they were, despite their very tragic ends.

My gut tells me that this is why my birthday has been my day of choice for good causes: a time when something positive could come out of the day designed to celebrate being alive another year. To lose a child on her birthday and to lose another child the day his own child was born had to be crushing for Grana. She had to be a block of granite to get through times of celebration with that kind of looming grief.

I hadn't self-diagnosed this connection in my story until I began thinking about writing this book. So many donors I met through this adventure had very surface-level explanations for choosing to give away their kidneys.


"It just made sense."

"It was the right thing to do."

"It was a no-brainer for me."

I can appreciate those sentiments. I can also appreciate the need to stay afloat on top of the water in the stories we tell. Diving into the deep end of our subconscious to explore how our brains really work and how our life experiences shape our souls can be scary. So yes, donating a kidney just made sense, but why did it make sense for you? No, really, why?

For me, childhood birthdays were always masked by balloons and cake. My dad and sister made sure of that. We celebrated the day as any other family would, with the bright side. But to celebrate a birthday indicates that one had to be born. Someone did the work to enable my existence, and it wasn't just my dad. In my life, that someone was missing from every single birthday I ever had, except the very first one.

Birthdays brought an invisible cloak of sorrow to me in a way that needed to be undone, somehow, someway. I chose to focus on the positive. That's why I gave things away: blood, hair, clothes, my kidney. I found a way to give birthdays a new meaning. A counterbalance to the grief I felt was there, but I couldn't really explain its presence until now.

Through encounters with other volunteers at IOPO, I found the community I never knew existed and never realized I needed. To hear folks talk about their loved ones who died too soon, particularly those who died by suicide, was something I could never appreciate. I was too conflicted, too sad, and too pissed to give breath to those feelings. Growing up, I would often get asked about my family, and then the next question would almost always be, "What happened to your mother?" If I told you I just magically appeared in the world one day in November 1976, would you change the subject already?

I eventually found the words and my voice to talk about my uncle because I knew him. I had stories to tell about him, and we had a pretty solid, but short, history. He cared for my sister and me. He was an avid comic book collector. He worked at the rubber mill and ate a lot of junk food. His death, while tragic, brought life to others. I was proud of him for that, and it stuck with me enough to change the trajectory of my own life and the life of my recipient in Pennsylvania.

The IOPO staff regularly had one of its volunteers attend and share their personal donation story with everyone at their monthly meetings. Marti reached out to me with an invitation to participate. I agreed and got the specifics to help me prepare. I'd be standing in front of a roomful of staff. I'd have ten minutes. I'd need to arrive by 11:00 a.m.

I had a few weeks to plan out my thoughts and build up the stamina to tell this newly elaborative personal story to a roomful of strangers. Except, this room wasn't filled with the typical stranger I was accustomed to. My story was deeply intermingled with their everyday work lives. It was the letter Grana received from IOPO that she tucked into every drawer in the house. It was their words and their deeds way back in 1990 that made it even possible for me to be standing in front of them. For them, it would be personal, and they didn't even know it yet. It was an opportunity for the IOPO staff to see how their work could affect people decades after the fact, and how it affected me in a major way.

That morning, I got in the car and made the drive down to Indianapolis. It was about three hours of road time for me, which was exactly what I needed to practice. I had to say the words, and I had to say them out loud as many times as I could before having to say them in front of an audience.

Aside from the workshop with Brianna, I hadn't yet verbalized those new words or my elaborated story. I hadn't put Uncle Ed's death and Grana's endurance out there into the universe in this way. I was able to write about these things, but could I say them without falling apart? Without needing someone to save me from the front of the room with tissues and a "there, there, dear?"

As I glanced at my notes, the words spilled out into the car. I could feel my throat constrict and my voice get choppy as I inched along. "It's probably the hardest decision a mother has to make, but my Grana set aside her grief for a moment and allowed my uncle to live on…" With each attempt at telling the story, I got a little further along before the tears emerged, before it got too hard to speak. By the time I made it to that parking lot in Indianapolis, the words flowed better, and the tears remained deep down inside. I was as ready as I was going to be.

Marti met me at the door and escorted me inside to the room full of organ procurement professionals. They smiled intently as Marti introduced me, and the room went quiet. What I said when I got up there, I don't exactly know. I knew what I wanted to say. I had just rehearsed it for three hours. But if my words came out as I intended them to, it is still a mystery. That is how my mind works sometimes; it switches to autopilot in times of stress.

I do remember the attentive faces staring back at me, though. I remember the tilt of the head, the smiles with the pursed lips, and the absence of air movement. There were no clicking noises from retractable pens. The silence was enormous and perhaps a necessary part of this kind of encounter. Everyone in that room knew what grief looked like, and it was staring them right in the face, doing her best not to turn into a puddle.

It was weeks later that I received the most encouraging email about my trip to Indianapolis. An IOPO staff person got my address from Marti and wanted to thank me for coming to talk with them. "Because of your story, I am looking at becoming a donor myself." I must not have bombed that one too badly. There's hope for me yet.

The *988 Suicide & Crisis Lifeline* provides emotional support for people in distress in the U.S. 24/7 via text, call, and chat services. No judgment, just help. Learn more at 988lifeline.org.

*The Trevor Project* is the leading suicide prevention and crisis intervention nonprofit organization for LGBTQ+ young people, providing information and support to LGBTQ+ young people 24/7, all year round. Learn more at thetrevorproject.org.

# Chapter 15

# I Donated a Kidney, Now What?

My earliest IOPO volunteer gigs began with Tim or Uncle Steve at my side and usually landed us at a senior citizens' health fair somewhere in the region. Telling my story in a compelling manner wasn't the primary motivator in these types of settings. Busting myths about donation was the mission at hand. Folks of a certain age who opposed donation often felt one of two ways about the matter: that their doctors would not try to save their lives if they knew they were planning to donate their organs when they died, or that, because they already had X or were diagnosed with Z, their organs were of no use to anyone upon death.

Being a mythbuster meant I had to have a certain level of credibility under my belt. I learned quite a bit through this experience myself, and the training at IOPO filled in the gaps. By being the niece of a donor and also being a living donor, who could disbelieve anything I had to say about this topic? Plus, Tim and Uncle Steve spoke from the perspective of actual recipients, so we covered all the bases.

Traditional college students were the ones I took an interest in. I thought they were at the right age to be daring and curious enough to consider living donation. I had a chance to test out that notion firsthand when Tim and I were offered the opportunity to take over a health class on a local university campus. It was an annual program that IOPO did through the college, and we were the lucky recipients of the task that year. I developed a PowerPoint presentation about donation, complete with the Katie Couric segment about kidney chains to play. Tim came fully prepared and ready with his recipient story.

We spent an hour and a half with the class and had a great discussion. After we talked about deceased donation, I asked them to consider what questions they would have if they were faced with the decision to donate a kidney right now. As I answered questions about costs, recovery time, and pregnancy, a few students became emotional. When I asked the class to raise their hands if they knew someone who needed a transplant, those students did so.

It didn't matter what room I found myself in; I often met people with this connection. People who kept this kind of grief to themselves, because there was little they could do about it anyway. While one person struggled to survive on the waitlist, the rest of the family were spectators, helplessly watching them deteriorate. That was the case with the students in the room that day. A year passed before I learned that one of those young people signed up to become a living donor. Perhaps Tim and I were the whisper she needed to hear that day, a helpful nudge of facts and experience that gave her the confidence.

IOPO's annual educational event, "Life is Cool," was a partnership with the local hospital that aimed to teach young people how to live a healthy lifestyle by taking care of their organs. The room was set up with display stations showcasing different parts of the body. Each group would have just a few minutes at each table to learn about the function of a specific organ before they moved on to the next one. Tim worked at the pancreas station, Uncle Steve at the lung station, and I was across the room at the kidney station, for obvious reasons.

My job, along with the rest of the volunteers in the room, was to appeal to a very energetic demographic: every single fourth grader in the county. As each school bus dropped off the kids, they bounced up the hospital stairs to learn about salt intake, touch a pig heart, try on eyeglasses, and more. Then, they all congregated in the middle of the room to hear from Dr. Mason about the dangers of smoking. They were at an impressionable age and had many good questions, which made the program very worthwhile. But there were hundreds of them, and by the end of the day, we were all exhausted.

The next day, *The Star* wrote an article about the event entitled "Area Fourth Grade Students Learn About Organ Donation.[50]" Above the article was a picture of a group of students at the kidney station and me. I was showing them how to properly remove their disposable gloves after touching the kidney on our table. I wonder just how many students would remember what I told them about salt intake versus how that kidney felt through their gloves.

As time went on, my volunteering evolved. I continued to participate in IOPO activities, but I was also invited to non-IOPO events throughout the region. Roxy, the tech at our Vet's office, asked me to speak at an awareness meeting she organized for her husband and his brother. "ShareLife" was the event she hoped would get the two of them off the waitlist and equipped with fully functioning living donor kidneys. I was tasked with talking to family members and friends about my experiences on the other side of the coin, hoping to address any questions or concerns they had about becoming donors.

To ensure I had the most up-to-date information about donating a kidney through NKR, I kept in communication with them. Shortly after my surgery, Diane had left the organization, but their finance person, Tom, responded to my email inquiries for brochures. I would tell him what I was up to, and he'd send me a stack of "Your Kidney is Waiting for You" brochures in the mail. It was my tool for engaging those who were serious about donating, and I tried to distribute them wisely.

My missing organ also got me into a few unexpected circles. I asked our family life insurance agent, Mike Johnson, to quote an increase in my policy. Considering life insurance companies were known to frown upon living donors, I was curious if that would be the case for me, too. I was the first client Mike had with this scenario, and he was intrigued by the whole situation as much as I was. A nurse came to collect blood and urine samples, and he came to complete the paperwork and to hear more about my donation. Then, he invited me to his Rotary Club meeting.

Mike filled the room with Rotarians and local funeral home directors. Not only did he arrange for a local reporter to attend, but the newspaper also featured my story on the front page of The Bryan Times,[51] and he came back with glowing reviews of my insurance evaluation. Turns out my policy had been upgraded due to my health. They concluded I had to be extremely healthy to give away a kidney; therefore, I would become a Premier policyholder with more coverage and lower premiums. Unfortunately, not every donor like me has the same policy outcome as I did. Why was this industry so cautious of us?

I found myself increasingly moved to talk about organ donation, and it seemed there was never a shortage of people interested in hearing about it. My story became fully fleshed out, and I could shorten or expand it depending on the mood of the room. I was able to verbalize the hard stuff, but not too much, because that remained emotional off-limits territory.

The labor movement was no stranger to having me participate in my new role as "neighborhood kidney donor" at their events, either. Typically, I would attend picnics and meetings to talk about trade and policy. My action calls would usually bring folks together to address the downward spiral of manufacturing jobs, but my portfolio had evolved. My voice appealed to the masses in a whole new way by offering them yet another opportunity to help each other.

As a member of the A. Philip Randolph Institute Chapter in Fort Wayne, an organization of black trade unionists and allies who fight for racial equality and economic justice, I also spoke at our regional conference. The program included a health component, and I was invited to share donation literature and information with attendees. Before my time with IOPO, I hadn't fully realized how race and ethnicity factored into waitlist demographics and the pattern of systemic racism that the data revealed.

Black Americans make up a disproportionate number of those on the waitlist and those who need transplants. According to Donate Life America:[51]

Black/African Americans, Hispanics, and Pacific Islanders are three times more likely to experience end-stage renal disease than Caucasians. Black/African Americans are three times more likely to progress to kidney failure than Caucasians. Hispanics are 1.5 times more likely to progress to kidney failure than the non-Hispanic population. 60% of those on the national transplant waitlist represent multicultural communities.

Our Northeast Indiana Labor Day Picnic at Headwaters Park was an ideal place for IOPO to have a presence and share information about donation with the thousands of folks who participated. I had had an informational booth there for several years to talk about manufacturing, and I knew IOPO would have a welcome ear. The IOPO booth was right next to mine, so that I could help them feel welcome in the new arena. Several IOPO volunteers came to talk about donation, including my pal Tim.

IOPO hoped to register a few new donors and reach a new demographic: good union people. Turns out, they registered so many donors during that one-day celebration that it set off a chain of invitations for IOPO to participate in other activities within the labor movement, from the Central Labor Council level down to the local union level. They even attended the biggest UAW event in the state, the Local 2209 Membership Picnic. Awareness was indeed blooming in the union.

With my consistent advocacy around donation, I was invited to attend the annual NKR Gala in New York each year. It became the place where I reconnected with my uber-committed and passionate surgeon, Dr. Milner, who was a member of the NKR Board and attended regularly. Through this avenue, I also built my family of donors. Finding donors like me was still a long shot in any room other than that fancy banquet hall with way too many forks on the table. It was nice to connect with more of them and to build camaraderie and connections for when we all went back to our home states. Ray Mueller, the donor I sat with our very first year, was also invited back. He owned a communications company for non-profits and volunteered his skills to record the Gala each year.

When it was time for NKR to develop donor testimonials for their outreach program, Ray and I were together again. He produced more than a dozen videos for NKR, which were very well done. His ten-minute productions, including the one of my story, have been seen hundreds of times.[52] Sure, there's little chance of them going viral, unless, of course, we were speaking through interpretive dance on a TikTok wearing flashy disco pants. There are no death-defying stunts or celebrity appearances in them either. But in the world of kidneys, all of Ray's videos are top-notch.

Through Josh Morrison, another donor I met at the NKR banquet, I was looped into the world of kidney legislative advocacy, which was right in my wheelhouse. He formed a non-profit called Waitlist Zero to advocate for greater support to increase living donor rates. One method was to get their message and their legislative efforts out into the media for curious readers to learn about donation. When the articles were published, it was time to react.

Waitlist Zero would receive inquiries from readers interested in becoming donors and learning more. They would then be connected with folks like me, willing to share how our donation experiences evolved. This would give curious people an idea of what they might expect if they decided to donate too. It was a way to connect a potential donor with a real person who had already done what they were considering doing. It was a way to build a movement of donors, one phone call at a time.

Through Waitlist Zero and its spin-off, the Coalition to Promote Living Kidney Donation, legislative work had been underway for years to support future donors financially and to develop a database to track our long-term health, something that wasn't being monitored by anyone, anywhere. One way to wrangle members of Congress into supporting an issue was to get them to join the club, by way of the Congressional Kidney Caucus.

At the time, I was quite familiar with the halls of Congress and the committee appointments of the Representatives. I even worked to bring attention to the Steel Caucus and the Buy America Caucus to ensure manufacturing initiatives were embraced. But I had no idea there was a caucus explicitly designed for those who were passionate about kidneys. That gave me an angle of focus. Appealing to a member of Congress to join a caucus seemed like an easy lift. When my work took me to D.C., I spent my free time walking from congressional office to congressional office, sharing that information.

Academia also recruited me to be one of its subjects. Whenever a university study emerged that amplified donors' voices, the request would find its way to me. I have participated in surveys and interviews on donor choice, donor pre-preparation, and donor motivations, among other topics. As my circle of donors expanded, so did my ability to bring others into the fold of these things. If I were invited to participate in a study, I would circulate the ask to dozens of others. Due to my kidney connections over the years, I had become a relied-upon resource.

By the middle of 2015, Mat and I were ready for a change in scenery. I needed a reset, and Mat was seeking more meaningful work. We both longed for a destination where the icicles didn't form on the inside of the windows. That summer, we set out on our new adventure in Los Angeles. Mat joined the team at the environmental non-profit, TreePeople, where he was the official "fixer of everything that was broken." He loved it, and it suited him perfectly. I, on the other hand, arrived in LA with a much different agenda than what I'd previously had.

I said goodbye to the hours on the road and said hello to an opportunity to spill the words onto paper. There would be no more frequent flyer miles or dinners alone in faraway hotels. There would be no more lobby reports or congressional meetings. I was officially clocking out. This kind of upheaval from someone so committed to the labor movement may seem a curious twist in this story you're reading. Why would someone like me choose to walk away from the movement I loved and the comforts of the direct deposit? For my own well-being and personal enrichment, it was time.

Being without a job meant I had all the time in the world to pour myself into my words. I had so much to say and share that I didn't want to miss my chance to tell the stories before I forgot them all. While the images were still fresh in my mind, I wanted to write about segments of my life. This book you're reading now was going to be the first item to check off my list. I was going to breeze through the chapters, typing a thousand words a minute. It would be published, and you'd see me at your local independent bookstore, signing copies and shaking hands. But then, the cancer came.

We were in LA for just six short months when Mat was diagnosed with Stage Four Squamous Cell Carcinoma. We were fortunate I had that newfound free time, so I could spend it learning how to help him through it. Since neither of us had first-hand experience with cancer in our family, we had an incredibly sharp learning curve. Two surgeries, six doses of chemo, and thirty-five rounds of radiation eventually got him on the road to recovery. And of course, all the nutrient-rich smoothies and magical soups I made. That year-long experience has been officially solidified in our minds as #ShitStorm2016.

As we focused on Mat and his well-being, I also sought connections in our new city to help us feel embedded in the San Fernando Valley. I officially joined a nearby Unitarian Universalist church after years of favorable visits to UU congregations and thought-provoking discussions with UUs across the country. Marti Cooper from IOPO, which eventually became known as the Indiana Donor Network (IDN), also happily introduced me to her counterparts at OneLegacy, the Los Angeles Organ Procurement Organization. The opportunities to connect were everywhere in our new city. I was bound to find "my people."

OneLegacy performed the same functions as the folks working with Marti at IDN, but because of the density in the LA region, they were huge and covered a lot of ground. Although they were responsible for organ, eye, and tissue donation for just seven counties surrounding Los Angeles, our 20 million people, 200+ hospitals, and eleven transplant centers made OneLegacy the largest organization of its kind in the world. And as I would soon find out, they had significant reach all around the globe.

The new ambassador volunteer training at OneLegacy was held in downtown LA. I was committed to driving as little as possible in our new city to counter the work mileage my body had endured. I took a bus, two trains, and walked the last mile to avoid traffic. The training was in a hotel with a selection of conference rooms. You know, the kind where thousands of people converge for events. The kind where you pay extra to park your car. We had just one room dedicated to us, but it was enormous enough to hold a concert for the likes of James Taylor. There was no circle of folks around a conference table like back in Indiana. Instead, dozens upon dozens of people were in that training with me, so much so that a giant chunk of time had to be allotted to do introductions.

It allowed me to hear my new peers' stories. They really weren't that different from those I heard in Indiana, except some of them came carrying signs or pictures of the people they'd lost or were there to celebrate. Some told of scripts or films they had in the works about their stories, which felt very appropriate considering we were in the heart of the entertainment industry.

But one group in attendance really challenged my ability to hold it together. You could tell by the way they were seated that they were a solid family unit. One by one, they stood up, some of them in tears, said their name and then their honored affiliation:

"My name is… and David Rodriguez was my uncle."

"My name is… and David Rodriguez was my brother."

"My name is… and David Rodriguez was my son."

"My name is… and David Rodriguez was my cousin."

It was heartwarming to see how the family of David Rodriguez came out in droves to honor him this way. It was also heartbreaking to see someone who was so loved by their family now gone. Donor family members, recipients, and caregivers were joined in that room in the same way they were in Indiana. There were just more of them.

As I became active in the OneLegacy Ambassador Program, I began meeting living donors who had been volunteering their time. I was excited to hear their stories and how they stumbled upon OneLegacy. Each of their histories varied, with most learning about OneLegacy through their recipients. With hundreds of ambassadors doing the good work in our region, there were twenty-five living donor ambassadors when I first joined the effort. Finding a connection there felt right to me. We belonged in these circles. But where were the rest of us?

Being an ambassador meant I'd regularly meet new people in "the family." I would sign up to volunteer at an event that interested me, and whoever else showed up would be my partner(s) for the day. It was a nice way to meet so many new people and to learn their donation stories in real time. We were all so different yet so intricately connected.

The variety of volunteer opportunities with OneLegacy was expansive. Given that many organizations were headquartered in LA, there were numerous fundraisers, galas, and networking events to attend to represent OneLegacy. There were also public speaking gigs at all the partner hospitals, where we would share our donation stories with new employees, nurses, or doctors. Then, there were other events complete with swimming pools and movie stars.

My willingness to talk about donation landed me in some fascinating places. I have been able to walk on carpets that were varying degrees of red. My wardrobe had to include a few things that resembled a "cocktail dress" for occasions when my black dress slacks would not suffice. To be in the same room as Boyz II Men, in Jane Seymour's backyard for a dinner party with her and other non-directed donors like me, to meet Lisa Simpson's saxophone player, and to share my kidney tales with the writers of the television series, New Amsterdam, all felt surreal. How regal had my very ordinary life become?

My volunteer efforts gave me a platform to share impactful information with the world. Had it not been for my pal Tim Musser, this community would have existed without me knowing about it. For donors like me without a Tim Musser in their lives, there had to be a way to streamline the introduction between donors and organ procurement organizations. All living donors should know that this community was waiting for them, right?

There wasn't yet an official home for people like me, a designated club where once you donated, you got your membership card. No, you had to find your people somehow and then find a way to fit into their programs. That takes a lot of gumption and may be nearly impossible for introverted donors. Plus, some, like me, may not know they fit right in with a cadre of people who celebrate life after death. This connect-the-dots, match-the-donor-with-the-organization mission needed an agent.

My feeling of isolation after donation, like I'd never meet people like me, was real. I felt alone in my experience, having done this completely unrelatable thing. As I met more and more donors, specifically non-directed donors, many said the same thing. It's lonely being the only one.

Ray and I had been discussing this issue for quite some time when we saw each other at the NKR Galas. Each year, we were in a roomful of non-directed donors. Still, we didn't have the opportunity to meet and connect with all of them in the confines of an elegant five-hour banquet with four forks, three glasses, two appetizer plates, and one perfect agenda. We thought about the possibilities that existed for mobilizing such a collection of donors from around the country. What could we do if given the chance and some good old-fashioned solidarity?

We reached out to Garet Hil and Joe Sinacore, the gala's lead organizer. Given the enormity of the space reserved for the gala and its corresponding educational symposium for the medical teams, surely there must be an extra room near the broom closet that Ray and I could use beforehand to network with donors, to host an open house. We could build an email list and share information about academic studies seeking subjects. We could have video conferences to keep in touch. We could motivate each other to share our donation stories. The possibilities were endless, we thought.

Through continued communications with the NKR leadership, we solidified our first annual NKR Donor Open House in 2018. Dean Pomerleau, an NKR donor from 2017, was also looped in to work in partnership with Ray and me. He represented all NKR donors on the NKR Medical Board and could share his role with those who attended the open house. Dean, Ray, and I planned to introduce the idea of staying connected, then build an email list of those who wanted to keep in touch.

Given the amount of helpful information we had to offer donors who were just entering our family, we agreed that a monthly newsletter would keep them engaged and offer ideas for becoming more active, if they chose to. My experience generating newsletters afforded me the role of editor, along with collecting pertinent information to share. That, coupled with Dean's monthly update from the NKR Medical Board, gave us something tangible for donors not only to read but also to promote their own advocacy work.

The effort to stay connected was sure to help donors feel less alone in the world. It would give them the inspiration to become active in their own communities and introduce them to organizations and programs they could join, such as their local organ procurement organization. If they had a notion, our newsletter and our collaboration as non-directed donors could bridge the gap between isolation and activism. It could bridge the gap between unicorns across the country.

Our 2018 NKR Donor Open House went exactly as we anticipated. The hotel meeting room was filled with non-directed donors from the past year, many of whom were meeting others like themselves for the first time. We also had some in the room who had become donors through their connection to "Donor to Donor." NKR donor Ned Brooks started that group to help those who needed kidneys to advocate and search for donors. He and other donors like him saw a way they could help by becoming kidney mentors. Donor to Donor later became the National Kidney Donation Organization (NKDO) with an expanded mission to unite us regardless of our physical proximity.

While we only had an hour, we began our official email list, exchanged names, and explained our hopes to stay connected and build a network to support each other. It was an exciting first meeting. Through the simple act of information sharing, we had the potential to inspire each other to do even more great things.

Each month, Dean would share his report from the medical board meeting, highlighting pertinent information donors would find interesting. At the same time, I collected and tagged academic studies, feel-good articles, and advocacy alerts that inquiring minds might want to know. I also highlighted organizations we should all know about, like our local organ procurement organizations and UNOS, for example.

Through my news aggregation, I became even more informed about the world of kidneys and what varying organizations and countries were doing. There were so many angles of interest to include in a two-page newsletter that I quickly ran out of space. Each month, any inspiring news I found that didn't fit went into the queue for an upcoming issue. As donors sent links to events they were hosting or to articles in which they were interviewed, our newfound organizing idea became a collective effort.

As I read through content to decide what made it into each newsletter, I discovered Dr. Abigail Marsh's groundbreaking work on empathy, psychopathy, and the motivations of organ donors. In an interview with CBS News, Marsh shared her findings on the amygdala, the part of the brain associated with empathy. Turns out the brains of psychopaths have a smaller amygdala than the average person, while the amygdala of altruistic kidney donors was about 8% bigger than average.[53] It made me wonder what degree of control I had over my decision to donate in the first place.

I had been in self-discovery mode, trying to understand why I made this decision, and pointing to several external factors as the culprit, from my work to my childhood to Uncle Ed. Could an internal factor, like the size of my brain, have exacerbated all those feelings of empathy to trigger this response? Much like my wonderment after having my kidney removed and not knowing if it was actually gone, knowing how big my brain was in comparison to the average person felt like something to put on the to-do list for the next time Parkview had a sale on brain scans. Shouldn't I feel the absence of my kidney? If my amygdala were bigger, shouldn't I feel that too?

I learned a lot about the intricacies of donor health, including my own, through this process. The National Kidney Foundation posted an article about a woman who experienced depression after donation.[54] The title "A Mother Triumphs Over Depression After Donating a Kidney" drew me in. As I read about Traci's post-transplant depression and her feelings of grief and anxiety, it took me back to the days and weeks after my own donation. My emotions were all over the place, and I had no idea why.

According to the article, post-transplant depression was an actual diagnosis. Donors were experiencing anxiety, depression, and other emotional issues after transplant, and it was essential to recognize the signs and focus on well-being. Years earlier, when I donated, that would have been helpful to understand. Perhaps few people knew about this in order to share. My post-transplant depression might have been genetic, passed down from my mother's post-partum depression as far as I knew. As I sat there reading the article, diagnosing myself with zero years of medical school experience, I knew it was one of those tidbits of knowledge this newsletter was destined to carry to the masses.

Chapter 16

# A Rose by Any Other Name

As my volunteering with OneLegacy expanded, so did my involvement in its programs. Education within hospitals, cities, high schools, and even the Department of Motor Vehicles; the programs were embedded into all the places that mattered. OneLegacy had jurisdiction over 203 cities, and all of them needed to know about eye, organ, and tissue donation, so I signed up for the task. As an ambassador to cities, my responsibility to each city I adopted was to be the face of the cause, to communicate with the city officials, invite them to our advocacy events, and speak at their city council meetings. Speaking to people about important stuff like this eventually became a breeze.

From the council chambers of Beverly Hills to Malibu, and even the tiny town of Bradbury with 1,000 residents, I took the mic and shared the importance of organ donation. After speaking, I was often invited to take a picture with the mayor. Other times, the attendees in the room would stop me on my way to my seat to tell me about a recipient or donor they knew. Still other times, there were ovations. Ovations always felt painfully awkward, but I was warming up to them with each speech I gave. It wasn't an ovation for me, I convinced myself. It was an ovation for the cause.

Doing the city ambassador work also helped me navigate my new region. For the events I couldn't ride the bus to, I had to concede being on the road for. That meant traffic. Los Angeles was an enormous city in its own right. Add in the 202 other cities, plus traffic, and every trip took three times as long as it should. If you made a wrong turn and went out of your way only to turn back around, you might as well go home because the day was spent. My distaste for traffic and being in the car met a point of compromise by my interest in doing the work. But finding my way across Southern California without losing my marbles was a lesson in geography and patience. Is South El Monte just South of El Monte? Why are there thirteen different ways to get to Cerritos?

Before my time with OneLegacy, I had very little knowledge about the Rose Parade. My experience watching it on New Year's Day depended on my remembering what time to catch it on TV. It wasn't until I became immersed in the float festivities as an ambassador that I understood the significance of OneLegacy and the responsibility they had to promote donation out into the world. To put it lightly, it was kind of a big deal.

OneLegacy was the lead organizer in the Donate Life America float. At the urging of Gary Foxen, an inspired lung recipient, OneLegacy laid the foundation for a float dedicated to donation in 2004, for all organ procurement organizations to build upon.[55] By the time I came on the scene, the Donate Life float, its national partners, and its corresponding events and activities had become a sophisticated machine.

Each year, the parade float was designed to incorporate dozens of organ recipients and living donors, seated on the float and walking alongside it. The float also carried floragraphs of deceased donors from around the country, made entirely of floral and organic materials. All the people representing the float were chosen by their sponsoring organizations. They wanted to share the unique stories that needed to be amplified. Deceased donors, living donors, organ, blood, and tissue recipients; the float was representative of whom we were celebrating for the whole world to see and be inspired by.

Given there were hundreds of us, the ambassadors were given a myriad of tasks as part of the annual event. Even though the float drove down Colorado Avenue on New Year's Day, there were organized festivities for several weeks leading up to it that needed to be tended to. People flew in from everywhere to join the meetings, banquets, and dinners. All of these people shared a bond. They were grieving and celebrating the gift of life, all at the same time.

Each year, the float's floor was filled with roses dedicated in honor or memory of someone. People from all pockets of the country bought roses and wrote personal tributes as an official component on the float. If they were local, those folks could place their dedicated rose directly on the float during an organized ceremony in the days leading up to the parade. If they weren't local, others in our circle did that on their behalf.

The float, fully draped in various flowers, nuts, seeds, and spices, did not transform into its majestic, meaningful design each year on its own. It took hundreds of volunteers and hundreds of pounds of organic materials to make it so. Cutting the flowers off the stems to dry, making the cinnamon and the navy beans stick to the skin of the drum, gluing the straw onto the beaks of the metal birds; volunteers did it all.

My first time as a float volunteer was rough. I did a terrible job of maintaining my composure and declared I would never do it again. The Rose Dedication Ceremony happened at night that year. People lined up to enter the tent to sign in and receive the rose they had ordered to personally place on the float. Hundreds were in line to honor the family member they had lost who became a donor or the donor who enabled them to live.

The assignment put me as the second person those folks saw as they made their way along to collect the roses and personal tributes. I passed out the cards, which let them know how to access their photos from the evening. That way, they could focus on the moment of tribute and leave the professional photo taking to our team. As the moms, adorned with pictures of their donor kids and grandkids, came through, the ugly crier in me came out. The ugly crier in me came out with every grieving face.

I switched assignments halfway through the evening and became the last person the "Rose Dedicators" saw before entering the large warehouse that held our float. I was tasked with walking with them from the tent to the warehouse entrance and sharing Rose Parade facts along the way. Facts and information, I could easily handle that without tears. Then, I closed our conversation with my own abbreviated elevator speech of how I was connected to organ donation.

In my second year as a float volunteer, I detoured away from the emotion-filled sign-in tent and worked inside the warehouse with the professional photographers. My role was to sequentially write down the names of those being photographed so that when we uploaded the photos onto the website, there was an organized way for individual photos to be located. I stood behind the camera next to the photographer. The people came to me and gave me their names, then they stood in front of the camera holding their rose. The float, in all its vibrance, was the backdrop.

On the day I volunteered as a photographer assistant, participants from one of the featured Donate Life stories were there. I didn't know their story at the time, but I knew it was unique. As they collectively made their way to our area, I could sense they were all connected. There were smiles and laughter, but also wet eyes and sorrow.

From the look in her eyes, she was a grieving parent, but I didn't follow sports for National Football League Pro Konrad Reuland's name to ring any bells. Dad watched sports throughout my childhood, so much so that I regularly use sports analogies that I don't fully understand. Still, I only knew the familiar-looking guy walking with Reuland's mother was in the Major League Baseball Hall of Fame thanks to Adam Sandler's hit song about Hanukkah.[56]

"Put on your yarmulke

It's time for Hanukkah

The owner of the Seattle Supersonic-ahs

Celebrates Hanukkah

O.J. Simpson: not a Jew

But guess who is? Hall-of-fame member Rod Carew (he converted)."

As we coordinated their seating along the side of the float, the sadness in the eyes of Reuland's mother really got to me. A baseball legend her son admired since childhood was alive and standing next to her as the recipient of his heart and his kidney. It was yet another time I envisioned my Grana seated in her place. Feeling joy in the gift but pain in the loss. How do parents do this so gracefully?

When I got home, I told Mat how, once again, my day as an ambassador weighed heavily. To witness so much sadness being held together with such composure was not easy. In his usual fashion, he pointed out the obvious.

"You volunteer with an organization that deals with death and grief, babe. What do you expect?"

Each year, OneLegacy chooses its float walkers, riders, and floragraph honorees primarily from its pool of ambassadors. There was a lengthy application process, multiple service requirements encompassing multiple programs, and an interview process with a corresponding process of elimination. The email invitations sent out encouraged all of us to apply. Yet it felt highly impossible.

Each year, I witnessed my donor and recipient ambassador pals being chosen as walkers and riders. Their excitement overflowed into the room as their names were announced during our annual conferences. Other ambassadors were selected to have the donor in their lives honored with floragraphs. That was yet another honorable moment to bestow upon donors who could not be there but absolutely needed to be celebrated and recognized.

My curiosity about how things work compelled me to learn more about participation on the Rose Parade float. I watched the videos and read the Donate Life float website to learn about its history. There was a page dedicated to each year's float participants, with pictures and a brief story of each person's connection. As I scrolled through the pages of float riders and walkers, I stumbled upon a familiar face and a familiar story. He was there!

Max Zapata rode on the Donate Life float in 2012.[57] His words on the website conveyed his hope of inspiring others to give as well. To see his story resurface in my life again felt intentional. The year I gave my kidney away because he inspired me was the year he was riding the Donate Life float, which I was now thinking about applying for. Was Max Zapata my kindred spirit?

Participating with the Donate Life float on New Year's Day, as it drove down the boulevard, seemed like an experience my curious mind was built for. I rarely passed up eclectic, intimidating adventures, unless they involved bungee jumping or spending a lot of money. To do so in the name of advocacy and outreach for organ donation made the idea even more appealing. I wouldn't have to travel very far, but I would have to set a dozen alarm clocks to wake up really early. That was a compromise I was willing to make.

The year I applied, I was a bit clunky. Having just a short term of OneLegacy volunteerism under my belt made me feel like an underdog to begin with. The application questions were easy to complete, but the corresponding documentation left me with more questions than answers. It's optional, but is it really? I submitted my paperwork on time and then moved on. If they chose me, great. If I were not chosen, all the better for an ambassador pal who was. There was no losing in this equation.

While my first attempt at walking alongside the Donate Life Rose Parade float ended with me watching it from my couch in my slipper socks instead, my second attempt took an entirely different turn. That time, I added all the recommended bells and whistles to my application. I submitted letters of recommendation along with my application. Harry and Pat were happy to write a letter of support for me on behalf of our now solidified kidney bond. Marti from the Indiana Donor Network also wrote a reference of all the work we did together to encourage donation in Indiana. I compiled a collage of photos from the various events I volunteered for with OneLegacy. It resembled a portfolio more than an application, and it did the trick.

I was called in for an official interview. Although I'd held dozens of jobs and volunteer gigs in my lifetime, I rarely fell victim to any procedural interview. I seldom had to proclaim anything to anyone sitting across the table from me, and I rarely had to lay myself vulnerable to anyone holding the cards. I had been incredibly privileged in my life to evade such traumatic experiences that many folks must regularly endure. This I know to be true. Preparing for this interview proved to be about as painful as I anticipated the interview itself to be.

"Tell us something you wouldn't want anyone to know" or "If you were a tree, what kind of tree would you be?" These were questions that came to mind that folks in the working world have been asked in interviews. My stomach turned as I thought of all the ways I might be expected to be thoughtful and poignant and all the ways I'd most likely fall on my face.

As I walked into the OneLegacy boardroom, I was greeted by Erika and Gavin, our volunteer coordinators. They, along with other OneLegacy staff, welcomed me and asked me to have a seat. What transpired in that boardroom, perhaps only the notetakers can fully recall. Like most of my stressful speaking experiences, my brain went into autopilot. I remember being asked whether I could handle the emotional toll of being in the spotlight and whether I was comfortable speaking to journalists and TV crews. But the rest, who knows?

Weeks later, Gavin and Erika called to let me know I was chosen to represent OneLegacy as the Float Walker for 2019. They congratulated me and told me to keep it quiet since the names of all the selected ambassadors were to be announced at our annual conference, which was still weeks away. I was unable to attend the conference, so I needed to create a 30-second video to share, thanking OneLegacy and expressing my excitement about being chosen.

Gavin said he was particularly moved in my interview when I told them, "I'm not special. Anyone could tell this story if they have the will to do it." That sounded exactly like how I felt. I'm glad that I didn't fall all over my words. My brain, on autopilot, instinctively knew exactly what to say. It was more proof I could trust it to pull the words out and toss them into the universe accordingly.

Our first activity related to the impending Rose Parade took place in October. It was our group photo opportunity, held at the Wrigley House in Pasadena. Many of us representing OneLegacy had our picture taken together and toured the historic house and grounds.

Our second activity was the joint Donate Life America and OneLegacy event, where they unveiled the partially assembled float and all its participants in mid-December. Called the "First Look Event," it was an opportunity for the press and the public to converge in a chilly, oversized warehouse to see the beauty of the float in its infancy. "Rhythm of the Heart" was our float name that year, symbolized by many musical instruments and drums from African cultures to emphasize the resemblance of a beating heart and the power of music to heal. Each local float participant was also announced, with our stories on display for the world to see and the press to report on.

Jolene Vargas was chosen as our OneLegacy recipient rider. She was a two-time kidney recipient who needed a third transplant due to the kidney disease she had lived with most of her adult life.[58] She was an all-around awesome person I had come to really love. We both lived in the valleys north of Los Angeles, so our volunteer paths crossed regularly. I valued our partnership at those events because she was very open about life as a kidney recipient. I learned a lot about the after-effects of donation from the other side of the donation table and could ask her anything.

Cathy Mora was selected as our Embajadora, representing our crucial Spanish-speaking volunteers within OneLegacy. Thirty-nine years prior, Cathy gave her kidney to her sister just three weeks after giving birth to her third child.[59] I had not volunteered with Cathy prior to the float festivities, but loved her energy and spirit.

The families of the OneLegacy floragraph honorees were also present to share the stories of their loved ones. Alexander Sonora, Dennis Brown, Dylan Stump, Erik Fitzpatrick, Jose Luis Cruz Jr., Francisco Esparza, and Josh Pearlman were our featured donors for 2019. The parents and siblings who joined us for the First Look Event were so proud of their loved ones for having saved so many lives, yet they were grieving inside for their absence. I, too, was grieving their absence. This environment was very difficult for me to maneuver within, wearing the frail armor of a highly empathetic person.

Shortly after the First Look Event, news reports began emerging from across the country featuring people chosen to participate in the Rose Parade. Sponsored by organ procurement organizations, transplant hospitals, blood banks —you name it —the stories were exploding. The Rose Parade was a big deal, and the press coverage reinforced that. I put my marketing hat on to see how I could help the cause with one more local story.

I reached out to Dave, the editor of *The Star,* back in Indiana. When I gave away my kidney in 2012, they put my donation story on the front page. Even though I relocated to Los Angeles, I thought, perhaps they'd still consider me a local. Maybe they'd squeeze a few words about the parade into the bottom fold under the hometown favorite Littlejohn Auction announcements or the "Nifty Under Fifty" classifieds section.

*The Star* reporter Kathryn Bassett called to interview me. She and I were in the same weightlifting class at the YMCA years ago, and I really liked her. She was intrigued by my story and asked a lot of good questions. I sent her photos of the recent First Look Event, with the float in the backdrop and the opening event at Wrigley House. There was no indication when the article would be published, so I sat back and hoped for the best.

Being chosen to represent OneLegacy in the Rose Parade had adjacent benefits. There were several events surrounding the parade meant to bring our donation family even closer together. With participants from all over the country, the receptions, meetings, and float-decorating opportunities helped solidify our collective bond. As a local participant, I was able to bring guests along for the festivities as well.

We first asked Harry and Pat to join us in Pasadena for the four days of events. Since they were now part of our family through our kidney bond, we thought they would most enjoy the experience. But traveling to Pasadena over the holidays requires taking out a large personal loan or selling the farm. Instead, Mat and I divvied up the tickets and invited our local friends based on what we thought they'd enjoy being a part of.

Mat and I checked into the Hilton Pasadena as scheduled. Although we lived about 20 miles away, it was best to stay as close as possible because holiday traffic would likely make it impossible to enjoy the whole schedule of events. With so many places to be and events to participate in, it would be easy to lose track and show up late or not at all. I hated to be late for anything and certainly didn't want to miss out. I was thankful Mat devoted all those days to being my right hand and most valued personal support.

With float participants from across the country flooding the hotel, it was exciting to see so many people representing their states and their donation programs. Even Kelli from the Indiana Donor Network was there to accompany two families whose loved ones were being honored with floragraphs. I tried to meet as many people and hear as many stories as I could, and I really absorbed the gravity of their experiences in a way I was trying to avoid. I found myself in tears often as I was listening to them talk about their loved ones who died and were being honored.

The hallways and meeting rooms were bustling with activity, either for us or by us. Pictures and stories of all the float honorees lined the lobby. Keychains and pom poms were piled high for anyone to take. Bryan Stewart, who had worked with the Donate Life float for years, had written a book about its history. He had a table set up outside the banquet room and was passing out signed copies of "Hope Blooms."

Mat, I, and our local friends immersed ourselves in the inspiring festivities and heartfelt events. It was a mosaic of meaningful experiences that I was privileged to be a part of. I was just a girl who watched the news and decided to do a thing, but there I was, encapsulated in this big new family who celebrated me as much as I celebrated them. And while I tried not to cry, I knew I was in the company of those who knew a good cry could make all the difference. It releases the storm to make room for the rainbow. I had to do a better job of acknowledging that.

In its special holiday edition on New Year's Eve, *The Star* again put yours truly on the front page, this time with Jolene by my side. "Riding with the Roses: Former Local Resident Promotes Organ Donation in Annual Parade" was the title of the article, which eclipsed half of the front page.[60] The article was a great addition to the collection of stories that highlighted the float and its significance in organ and tissue donation outreach that year. All told, through 1,200 media stories, 600 million people were reached by the Donate Life float and the donation message during that time period. Six hundred million "Media Impressions" is what they call it.[61]

The last Donate Life America event leading up to the parade was a big New Year's Eve celebration. All the honorees and their guests were invited to cut loose, with dancing and mingling, to celebrate the final phase of an inspiring and emotional experience. Sparkling beverages and tiny plates of crackers and cheese filled the room. Glasses and top hats with "2019" displayed in glitter were everywhere. A photo booth solidified the night with a memento for the road.

It was during this final celebration that I honored my Grana one more time for being such a major influence in my being in the room that night. Having her pearls around my neck and the dress she wore to marry, according to her, the "best" of her five husbands, was my way of bringing her to the ball. Through her stories of Uncle Ed, Grana was my ticket into that room. She was honoring her son through stories that kept him alive in her mind, and very much alive in mine. Her emerald green sloping neckline gown hung on me like I was a coat rack, but that didn't stop me from wearing it, the first time as I gave her eulogy and the second time that night, to honor her for being a genuine class act all my life.

Due to our early morning parade start, it was decided to celebrate the New Year on East Coast time rather than Pacific time, so we could all adjourn to get some sleep before our big reveal. I'm sure the organizers could predict there would be little sleep that night as anticipation climbed for the five-mile parade route and all the emotions that would overflow because of it. The 3:00 a.m. alarm sounded just two hours after I finally fell asleep. But I wasn't groggy. I was full of adrenaline for what was about to commence.

# Epilogue

On New Year's Day 2019, 700,000 people watched the Rose Parade in person as it made its way through the 5 ½ mile stretch of the city of Pasadena with Grand Marshal Chaka Khan leading the way. It was televised to more than 56 million viewers in the United States and an additional 28 million in 174 other countries. The Donate Life float, *Rhythm of the Heart,* received the distinguished *Judges Award* for most outstanding float design and dramatic impact.[62]

After the Rose Parade festivities of 2019 subsided, I got intentional about putting my thoughts on this kidney adventure into words. Based on one of my earliest elevator pitches written for speaking to hospital staff, a twelve-chapter outline emerged as my starting point for what these pages have become. As I scrolled through my old emails with Loyola and NKR, the brochures and paperwork, and the pictures from all of the meetings, events, and memorable moments of this period of my life, I knew I had a valuable message to share.

My goal of sharing this story is multifold. Not only did I want to share the message that regular folks like me can do impactful things when an opportunity presents itself, but also to recognize that what drives us to act and react can help us understand ourselves better. Our lived experiences help shape how we exist in the world and inform us of how we can meaningfully come into the lives of others, by chance or entirely on purpose.

I didn't fully grasp what it was that compelled me to jump into this decision until I lay myself down on that cold leather couch of self-assessment and began to dig in. If the act of non-directed donation were such a "no-brainer," as many say it is, there would be more of us in the world. Understanding what those influential pockets of time were for me was important for comprehending what drew me in. It piqued my curiosity as to what rationale might move others to take a similar plunge. Can people do big things without there being a root cause, without eventually coming face to face with the "why?" Perhaps, but I don't think so.

Grana told stories to share her love for her kids with our family. I kept those morsels close to my heart until Katie Couric reached into my living room that fateful November evening and summoned me to act. Grana never shared her memories in any official capacity, as I have with Indiana Donor Network and OneLegacy, and neither did any of our other family members. Why I became the spokesperson for our family's donation legacy may have more to do with the privilege I have been afforded than anything else. Available time and a platform are not readily accessible to everyone.

What happens when we lose the people we love is complicated. Some choose to channel that grief and pain into public pronouncements and celebration. Others prefer to hold that sorrow close and let it lie heavy on their hearts. I recognize and acknowledge that this emotional rollercoaster has occurred within me throughout my life, as far back as I can remember.

The same choices apply for living donors as well. Some donors wish to remain completely anonymous to the world, with very few people knowing of their deed. Others want to shout from the peak of Mount Kilimanjaro, "YES YOU CAN DO IT TOO," to inspire others to leave the world better than it was found. I slowly and awkwardly found myself in this camp of donors once I realized that my silence could prevent others from living their best lives. My inability to talk about myself had to take a back seat to the cause.

Discovering that the donation community was mobilized for advocacy was something I never anticipated. Making connections over grief and advocating for life alongside equally passionate people felt like a new frontier. Very much like discovering water in a desert, it never occurred to me that such an oasis existed. I did not expect to build the relationships I have over the years simply because I said "YES" to donation and then volunteered to talk about it.

The exact recipe that caused me to react the way I did after watching a ten-minute Katie Couric news segment remains a mystery. I was paying attention and believed I could help. I had Oprah reminding me, "Once you know something, you can't unknow it." I had Grana's whisper in my ear. I had Uncle Ed's legacy. My experiences in the labor movement and in my advocacy for justice intersected with this perfect storm, leading me to make a decision that allowed me to help in a way I never knew I could. To be of use in a whole new way.

Becoming a donor is the most neighborly thing we can do for each other. Many people have donated organs, but there are still not enough of us to end the waitlist. I long for the day when there are more donors than the need requires. Until then, may our curiosity and wonder continue to lead us toward wholeness, and may we find inspiration and comfort in the stories of others.

"Let it stew," as Grana would say. "Just let it stew."

# Afterword

by J. Randy Johnson,
Author of *Forced Reckoning*

When Rachel asked me to provide an afterword for her book, I was thrilled and overwhelmed as to what a good afterword should contain. Research helped provide ideas and thoughts, but in the end, it is meant to supplement the main content of the story. With that in mind, I realized there is more to share about Rachel, the author and exceptional human being, and how I came to know her.

I first met Rachel while she was employed by the United Steelworkers Union (USW) in Pittsburgh. We both worked in the Strategic Campaigns Department, and I was asked to mentor her in providing training courses and assistance to local unions. My career background with the union began when I was hired at a paper converting facility in 1986, and I honed contract bargaining skills. In 1996, I became a full-time union campaign staffer and did this until my retirement in 2014. During this time frame, three large union mergers required additional training for these members. Many new staffers were needed to conduct the essential training, Rachel being one of them.

Rachel was a very quick study and became fully engaged in providing members with much-needed support. In a brief period of time, she was ready to co-facilitate our union's training programs and prepare members for bargaining with their employers for better wages and improved safety and health conditions. In our line of work, this is known as a contract campaign.

One such contract campaign supports a national bargaining agreement for all union members in a particular industry nationwide. To negotiate a national agreement, we empower local members, typically by bringing them developed programs created by staff in our department. The most used program was called *Building Power,* in which local members worked together to develop a strategy and an action plan to build unified power in solidarity. Union members are always stronger together. And when left to their own devices, they come up with fantastic ideas that can really surprise employers.

One of these Building Power trainings that Rachel and I co-led was in support of the national bargaining agreement for members in the oil industry. We provided a three-day program to refinery workers in Lima, Ohio (and yes, there is an oil refinery in Lima). Everything was going as planned until day two, when I felt a slight pain in my chest. At my request, Rachel stepped up and finished leading the sessions so that I could rest.

We returned to our hotel later that evening with plans to meet for dinner. What I didn't know at the time was that I was experiencing symptoms of a heart attack. To put it mildly, it is not a pleasant experience. I called Rachel, and she drove me to the local hospital, where I suffered a major heart-stopping cardiac event. Because Lima, Ohio, has a heart center in its hospital, they were able to save my life quickly.

I call Rachel my hero for getting me to the hospital, sitting with me, contacting my spouse, and informing my colleagues. She was not done yet, as late that evening, she prepared to lead the class of oil workers on their final day of Building Power training by herself. The hardest session in the training program is the final day, where members develop the plan for their local union and coordinate it with a nationwide strategy. The local union officers who stopped by my hospital room that evening informed me of the wonderful job she did.

Throughout her book, Rachel explains incredible acts of courage and resilience with such humility. Even her description in Chapter 8 of this very event in Lima, Ohio, is not told from the perspective of someone who has something to prove. In whatever way she is asked to respond, she doesn't hesitate. I know she cringes when I call her my hero, but she'll always hold a special place in my life's story. Rachel has taken the lessons of the union —solidarity, fellowship, and justice — and has made them her life's purpose. So, am I surprised she donated an organ and authored this book? Not at all.

I reflect on my own family's life-saving organ donation story as I read Rachel's. My brother had suffered from liver failure for two years, but through the generosity of a family member, who became his living donor, he is alive and well today. I currently display a decal on my vehicle that reads "Donate Life, Recipient Family," with the same pride I see in Rachel, as a member of a donor family and as a donor herself. Rachel's story is a road map to the value of human life, and her compassion is beyond belief.

The world needs more Rachels in it.


J. Randy Johnson
Author, *Forced Reckoning*

# Discussion Questions

1. Why do you think the author wanted to tell their story? What do you think is the main message they wanted you to come away from reading the memoir with?

2. How, if at all, did this memoir relate to your own life? Did it evoke any memories or connections for you?

3. Did the memoir change your opinion or perspective, or did it confirm or contradict any of your assumptions or expectations about organ donation, altruism, or the notion of justice?

4. How did the author portray the other people in their life? What was their influence or impact on the author's life choices or outcomes?

5. What are some of the ethical, moral, or social implications in the story? How does it challenge or support your own values or beliefs?

6. Reflecting on Chapter 7, would you have answered any of the doctor's questions differently from the way the author did?

7. What factors impacted the choices the author made? Do you think these factors reflect what it's like in the world today? What makes you say that?

8. With Chapter 12 in mind, if you were to write your own letter to an organ recipient, living donor, or donor family member, what would it say?

9. Did you highlight or bookmark any passages from the memoir? Did you have a favorite quote or passage? If so, share which and why?

10. How would you adapt this memoir into a movie? Who would you cast in the prominent roles?

11. If you could ask the author one question about this book, what would it be? Answers await: rachel@bennettsteury.com

# Acknowledgements

This book has been a long time coming. It took a lot of love and effort from many people for this memoir to reach the library nearest you. Some days the words flowed like a waterfall, and other days they had to be vigorously shaken from my fingertips. Thankfully, here we are.

Through this memoir, I seek to honor my uncle. Uncle Ed saved the lives of five people through organ donation and healed countless others through his tissue donation. His memory and his contributions to a more just society have been a blessing to many. Thank you, Sam and Yvonne, for giving me the grace to tell our family story.

I am thankful to have discovered my publisher and its founder, Brenda E. Cortez, through the same organ donation circle I write about in this memoir. Having my story published under the BC Books imprint brings this long-running project full circle. We seek to support each other in this community through our deeds, our words, and our publications.

Because of my union, the United Steelworkers, I was able to see a project like this to its successful conclusion. I've had the privilege of working for and being a product of the labor movement, where family-supporting wages and benefits were foundational to providing opportunities to live meaningfully within and beyond the factory walls. As my friend, trade unionist Ed Sadlowski, used to say, "There's more to the good life than just turning a paycheck." I couldn't agree more.

Contributions from my esteemed colleagues helped to bookend my story in what I see as a perfect fusion of my life during that time. Thank you to the founder of the National Kidney Donation Organization (NKDO), living donor Ned Brooks, for writing the Foreword and recognizing the differences and the similarities in the stories donors tell. NKDO has been instrumental in offering living donor education, support, and mentorship, and I am proud to have participated in various projects and campaigns alongside the group since its inception. I am equally thankful to fellow author and trade unionist, J. Randy Johnson, for writing the Afterword to this memoir, revealing one of the most life-altering on-the-job experiences we've both had. I was fortunate to have been partnered with such an integral member of the United Steelworkers Strategic Campaigns Department in our field work supporting union education programs across the country.

As with every wild idea I have ever had, my much better half, Mathew Steury, has always been willing to help me make it happen. I typically start off by saying "I have an idea," at which time he takes a breath and holds on, as he never can predict what I'm about to propose. Once I declare with absolute certainty an eventual success, he nods, and we get to work. Thank you for loving me through this and everything. You are the mac-n-cheese to my peas, baby.

The development of the book cover was a dream team effort. Thank you to Meghan Hasse, who captured my silhouette during an interview many years ago and is a fitting representation for how I prefer to see myself: in the shadows. Unwavering admiration goes to Mat, who developed and refined all of the initial images and got our layout on the cusp of the finish line. I extend immense appreciation to the Cawley siblings for their creative tenacity: artist Georgia Cawley, who offered feedback and introduced us to graphic designer Brad Cawley-Hamm, who took our vision and perfected it into our final cover.

I want to honor and recognize my Massachusetts friend Beth Berry for being the very first person to read, review, and offer feedback on every single story, report, or case study that has been important to me, including this memoir. Your support was incredibly instrumental. Thanks to my test readers for their honest insight on this topic within my short stories, my website, and the contents of this memoir: Ned Brooks, Dan Cragen, Harry Dacanay, Randy Johnson, Rita Johnson, Yvonne Place, Denning Powell, Sarah Ramon, Jay White, and Megan White.

Thank you to the exceptional Helene Atwan for sound publishing guidance early on as I waded through the intricacies of the industry, and to my friend Terry Lowman for making the introduction. To actor, author, and friend Joyce Fidler, thank you for kick-starting my engine when I felt like throwing in the towel. Unitarian Universalists near and far have really united around this effort, and I appreciate you all for it.

Thank you to everyone at OneLegacy, Indiana Donor Network, Loyola Medical Center in Maywood, the National Kidney Registry, the National Kidney Donation Organization, the United Steelworkers, and the Alliance for American Manufacturing, who read all or part of my manuscript and gave me the thumbs up to keep writing.

To every reader of The Real Rachel BS newsletter on Substack who offered encouragement along the way via the myriad of feedback: you really know how to make a writer feel special.  #TeamSubstack: immense appreciation goes to our Founding and Sustaining members who helped fund this project: Joe Barry, Beth Berry, Joanne Leilani Carpenter, Shannon Catalano, Yujuan Chen, Georgia Cawley, Nalani Feliciano, Joyce Fidler, Greg Golden, Lynn Higashi, Beth Hollis, Ava Howard, Mark Kassis, Bob Kuznar, Shari Kuznar, Dennis Leazier, Lenley Lewis, Chris Long, Terry Lowman, Christina Mathers, Miles Okumura, Carol Plummer, Denning Powell, Stephen Schneider, Andy Schultz, Megan Schultz, Qining Sun, Rich Suter, Nicole Thibideaux, LaTreco Thompson, Shonda Thompson, Paula Tubert Golden, Jim Wallis, Eve Weinbaum and Becky Zimmerman. And to my Illinois friend and fellow SOAR member, Jeff Rains, who mailed me a twenty-dollar bill to reserve a signed copy of this memoir five years before publication, thank you for believing in me!

To my sister, Dara Bowen, and my dearest friend, Shonda Thompson, who were personally responsible for most of the happiest memories I have of growing up: you were the lighthouses to my lost kayak. Thank you for never wavering. To Dad, who, as a single parent, had to make a lot of life choices I'm sure he didn't want to, thank you to you, Grana Barb, Aunt Dove, and Grandma Rose for keeping Dara and me alive and loving us through life's curveballs. And finally, BIG MAHALO to our extended family in Hawaii, California, and the Midwest for all the support through the good times and bad.

To the inspirational writers who were in my life long before I knew who I was and loved me anyway: Teresa Lopez, Jason Martinek, Catherine Mulder, and Shonda Thompson, thank you.

To our housesitting community across the planet: appreciation goes to our clients for trusting us to care for all that they love. Every couch and every furry face I had access to was further inspiration to develop my craft.

I am grateful for the public library system because I had no idea how to do any of this before using its resources. The Gale courses I took to learn how to prepare a manuscript for publication, and the Ask a Librarian feature connecting me with knowledgeable professionals, were very helpful.

Finally, to the organ donation community, thank you for welcoming me in as one of your own and for inspiring me to share our story on these pages. I am so fortunate to have kidney recipient Harry Dacanay and his family in my life and as part of my family. I'm so grateful to have found you all.

# Web Resources

Author webpage https://www.bennettsteury.com/

OneLegacy Donate Life Float https://onelegacyfloat.org/

National Kidney Registry https://www.kidneyregistry.com/

The National Kidney Donation Organization https://www.nkdo.org/

The United Steelworkers https://usw.org/

To learn more or to register your organ donation decision, visit the Donate Life America website at https://www.registerme.org/

The 988 Suicide & Crisis Lifeline provides emotional support for people in distress in the U.S. 24/7 via text, call, and chat services. No judgment, just help. Learn more at https://988lifeline.org/

The Trevor Project is the leading suicide prevention and crisis intervention nonprofit organization for LGBTQ+ young people, providing information & support to LGBTQ+ young people 24/7, all year round. Learn more at https://www.thetrevorproject.org/

# Works Cited


ABC7 Chicago. (2010, March 31). *Loyola Hosts 1st Ill. Kidney Transplant Chain.* Retrieved July 10, 2019, from ABC7 Chicago: https://abc7chicago.com/archive/7359142/

Anderson, B. (2010, June 26). *Clovis Man's Kidney Donation Spurs 20 More.* Retrieved from The Fresno Bee: https://www.fresnobee.com/news/local/community/clovis-news/article19505739.html

Andrews, M. A. (2002, April 22). *How can you live without one of your kidneys?* Retrieved January 29, 2020, from Scientific American: https://www.scientificamerican.com/article/how-can-you-live-without/

Annette M. Jackson, PhD, D., & Kraus, MD, E. (n.d.). *Blood Tests for Transplant.* Retrieved January 5, 2022, from National Kidney Foundation: https://www.kidney.org/atoz/content/BloodTests-for-Transplant

Bassett, K. (2013, April 3). Area Fourth Graders Learn About Organ Donation. *The Star.*

Bassett, K. (2018, December 31). "Riding with the Roses Former Local Resident Promotes Organ Donation in Annual Parade". *The Star*, p. 1.

Board, K. N. (2013, Jan 31). *The year in stories.* Retrieved February 2022, from KPC News: https://www.kpcnews.com/news/latest/eveningstar/article_4102a7b3-c845-5167-a758-6017753cfd06.html

CBS Evening News with Katie Couric. (2010, November 10). Kidney Chains Link Total Strangers Saving Lives. CBS News. Retrieved from https://www.cbsnews.com/news/kidney-chains-link-total-strangers-saving-lives/

CBS News. (2019, July 8). *Scientists Studying Brains of Altruistic Kidney Donors Who Give Organs to Strangers.* Retrieved September 2025, from CBS News: https://www.cbsnews.com/news/kidney-transplant-donor-scientists-study-brains-of-altruistic-donors-who-give-their-organs-to-strangers/

Cuda-Kroen, G. (2012, July 2). *Organ Donation Has Consequences Some Donors Aren't Prepared For.* Retrieved August 19, 2019, from National Public Radio: https://www.npr.org/sections/health-shots/2012/07/02/155979681/organ-donation-has-consequences-some-donors-arent-prepared-for

Cullis, C. (2013, August 3). Kidney Donations Form a Chain of Life. *The Bryan Times*, p. 1.

Donate Life America. (n.d.). *Donate Life America.* Retrieved January 30, 2026, from Donate Life America: https://donatelife.net/donation/statistics/

Donate Life America. (n.d.). *Race, Ethnicity & Donation.* Retrieved July 2025, from Donate Life America: https://www.donatelife.net/race-ethnicity-and-donation/

Donate Life Rose Parade Float. (2011). *2012 Float Rider Max M. Zapata.* Retrieved June 12, 2020, from Donate Life Rose Parade Float: https://www.donatelifefloat.org/prod/components/media_center/float_riders/mzapata.html

Donate Life Rose Parade Float. (2018, December 1). *2019 Jolene Vargas.* Retrieved June 22, 2020, from Donate Life Float: https://www.donatelifefloat.org/wp/2019-jolene-vargas/

Donate Life Rose Parade Float. (2018, December 1). *2019 Catalina "Cathy" Mora.* Retrieved June 22, 2020, from Donate Life Float: https://www.donatelifefloat.org/wp/2019-catalina-mora/

Fehrman-Ekholm, I. E.-G., & Groth, C.-G. (1997, October 15). Kidney Donors Live Longer. *Transplantation*, 976–978. Retrieved May 21, 2019, from Transplantation: https://journals.lww.com/transplantjournal/Fulltext/1997/10150/KIDNEY_DONORS_LIVE_LONGER1.7.aspx#print-article-link

Goldfarb DA, M.S. (2001, December 1). Renal Outcome 25 Years After Donor Nephrectomy. *Journal of Urology*, 2043-2047. Retrieved May 21, 2019, from Journal of Urology: https://www.auajournals.org/doi/full/10.1016/S0022-5347%2805%2965502-4

Graham, J. (2010, March 10). *5 Good Samaritans Start Chains of Life.* Retrieved January 28, 2019, from Chicago Tribune: https://

www.chicagotribune.com/living/ct-xpm-2010-03-30-ct-met-kidney-transplant-20100330-story.html

Gunnerson, T. (2018, December 1). *A Mother Triumphs Over Depression After Donating a Kidney.* Retrieved May 21, 2020, from National Kidney Foundation: https://www.kidney.org/newsletter/patient-story-post-transplant-depression

Henderson, A. J., Landolt, M. A., McDonald, M. F., Barrable, W. M., Soos, J. G., Gourlay, W., . . . Landsberg, D. N. (2003, February 26). The Living Anonymous Kidney Donor: Lunatic or Saint? *American Journal of Transplantation, 3*(2), 203-213.

Ilana Silver Levine, L., & Marian Charlton, R. C. (2010, November). *Living Donors Overview.* Retrieved April 10, 2019, from National Kidney Registry: https://www.kidneyregistry.org/living_donors.php#myths

Kesner, J. (2009, February 11). *How a gift of a kidney transplant in California has linked New Yorkers.* Retrieved January 15, 2019, from New York Daily News: https://www.nydailynews.com/life-style/health/gift-kidney-transplant-california-linked-new-yorkers-article-1.393029#ixzz0p02VvzJg

Khidekel, M. (2010, February 23). *Organ Donation: How Christina Saved 11 Lives.* Retrieved January 25, 2019, from Glamour: https://www.glamour.com/story/organ-donation-how-christina-saved-11-lives

Lehman, O. (2012, August 18). Woman Donates Kidney to Stranger. (D. Kurtz, Ed.) *The Star*, p. A1.

Lotus, J. (2011, April 27). *River Forest Doctor One of Seven Loyola Staffers Who Have Donated Kidneys.* Retrieved July 9, 2019, from Wednesday Journal: https://www.oakpark.com/News/Articles/4-27-2011/River-Forest-doctor-one-of-seven-Loyola-staffers-who-have-donated-kidneys/

Loyola University Health System. (2010, July 1). *Loyola's Pay-It-Forward Kidney Program Pays It Forward For Wife of Chicago Police Officer.* Retrieved July 10, 2019, from NewsWise: https://www.newswise.com//articles/loyolas-pay-it-forward-kidney-program-pays-it-forward-for-wife-of-chicago-police-officer

M. Stadtler, B. S. (2005, November 3). The Donate Life Rose Parade Float: How an innovative, integrated public awareness campaign effectively reaches a worldwide audience. *European Transplant Coordinators Organization, Organs and Tissues*, 169-172. Retrieved June 12, 2020, from https://www.donatelifefloat.org/wp/wp-content/uploads/2015/06/110105_ETCOOrgansAndTissues_DonateLifeFloat.pdf

Milliman Inc. (2008). *Milliman Research Report 2008 U.S. Organ and Tissue Transplant Cost Estimates and Discussion.* Retrieved April 8, 2019, from Wayne State University Department of Economics: http://www.econ.wayne.edu/agoodman/7550/Week8/Previous/2008%20Milliman%20Report.pdf

Milliman Inc. (2011). *Milliman Research Report 2011 U.S. Organ and Tissue Transplant Cost Estimates and Discussion.* Seattle: Milliman Inc. Retrieved April 10, 2019, from http://us.milliman.com/uploadedFiles/insight/research/health-rr/2011-us-organ-tissue.pdf

Milliman Inc. (2014). *Milliman Research Report 2014 U.S. Organ and Tissue Transplant Cost Estimates and Discussion.* Seattle: Milliman Inc. Retrieved April 10, 2019, from http://us.milliman.com/uploadedFiles/insight/Research/health-rr/1938HDP_20141230.pdf

Milliman Inc. (2017). *Milliman Research Report 2017 U.S. Organ and Tissue Transplant Cost Estimates and Discussion.* Seattle: Milliman Inc. Retrieved April 10, 2019, from http://us.milliman.com/uploadedFiles/insight/2017/2017-Transplant-Report.pdf

Milliman Inc. (2020). *Milliman Research Report 2020 U.S. Organ and Tissue Transplants: Cost Estimates, Discussion and Emerging Issues.* Retrieved December 2021, from Milliman Inc.: https://www.milliman.com/-/media/milliman/pdfs/articles/2020-us-organ-tissue-transplants.ashx

Milliman Inc. (2025). *Milliman Research Report 2025 U.S. Organ and Tissue Transplants: Estimated Costs and Utilization, Emerging Issues, and Solutions.* Retrieved July 2025, from https://www.milliman.com/en/insight/2025-us-organ-and-tissue-transplants-costs-utilization

National Kidney Foundation. (2019). *Six-Step Guide to Protecting Kidney Health.* Retrieved January 15, 2019, from National Kidney Foundation: https://www.kidney.org/atoz/content/sixstepshealthprimer

National Kidney Registry. (2009, May 14). *Kidney Transplants Facilitated by a National Registry Can Save $100 Billion in U.S. Healthcare Costs White Paper draft version 8.1.* Retrieved April 5, 2019, from National Kidney Registry: https://www.kidneyregistry.org/pages/p223/White_Paper.php

National Kidney Registry. (2019). *NKR News Articles.* Retrieved from National Kidney Registry: https://www.kidneyregistry.org/pages/c1/in_the_news

National Safety Council. (2019, May 21). *What Are the Odds of Dying From..* Retrieved May 21, 2019, from National Safety Council: https://www.nsc.org/work-safety/tools-resources/injury-facts/chart

Nutt, A. E. (2010, January 19). *Chain of Life- Kidney transplant chain helps six patients.* (T. S. Ledger, Ed.) Retrieved January 15, 2019, from New Jersey Real Time News: https://www.nj.com/news/index.ssf/2009/06/kidney_donation_chain_of_life.html

OneLegacy. (2019, January 1). *2019 Donate Life Rose Parade Float Inspires Millions With the Powerful Message of Organ, Eye, and Tissue Donation.* Retrieved March 12, 2025, from BusinessWire: https://www.businesswire.com/news/home/20190101005046/en/2019-Donate-Life-Rose-Parade-Float-Inspires-Millions-With-the-Powerful-Message-of-Organ-Eye-and-Tissue-Donation

OneLegacy Foundation. (2019). *2020 Donate Life Rose Parade Float Campaign Sponsorship Opportunities.* Retrieved December 8, 2020, from Donate Life Float: https://www.donatelifefloat.org/forms/sp20/lib/sponsorships.pdf

Organ Procurement and Transplantation Network. (n.d.). *Donors Recovered in the U.S. by Donor Type Since 1988.* Retrieved January 26, 2026, from U.S. Department of Health & Human Services: https://optn.transplant.hrsa.gov/data/view-data-reports/national-data/

Organ Procurement and Transplantation Network. (n.d.). *How Organ Allocation Works*. Retrieved January 16, 2019, from Health Resources and Services Administration: https://optn.transplant.hrsa.gov/learn/about-transplantation/how-organ-allocation-works/

Organ Procurement and Transplantation Network. (n.d.). *Kidney Donors Recovered in the U.S. by Donor Type*. Retrieved January 26, 2026, from U.S. Department of Health & Human Services: https://optn.transplant.hrsa.gov/data/view-data-reports/national-data/

Organ Procurement and Transplantation Network. (n.d.). *OPTN Transplant Information Database Current U.S. Waiting List Candidates*. Retrieved January 26, 2026, from Department of Health and Human Services: https://optn.transplant.hrsa.gov/data/view-data-reports/national-data/

Sandler, A. (1996). *AZLyrics*. Retrieved June 12, 2020, from The Chanukah Song Lyrics: https://www.azlyrics.com/lyrics/adamsandler/thechanukahsong.html

Saulnier, B. (n.d.). *The Strongest Link*. Retrieved January 15, 2019, from Cornell Alumni Magazine: http://cornellalumnimagazine.com/the-strongest-link/

Singer, P. (2006, December 17). *What Should a Billionaire Give – and What Should You?* Retrieved April 3, 2019, from The New York Times: https://www.nytimes.com/2006/12/17/magazine/17charity.t.html

Singer, T., & Lamm, C. (2009). *The Social Neuroscience of Empathy*. (N. Y. Sciences, Ed.) Retrieved March 10, 2025, from Greater Good Science Center: https://greatergood.berkeley.edu/images/uploads/Singer_2009.pdf.

Sit, D. L. (2015, April). *Suicidal Ideation in Depressed Postpartum Women: Associations with Childhood Trauma, Sleep Disturbance, and Anxiety*. Retrieved March 16, 2022, from National Center for Biotechnology Information, U.S. National Library of Medicine: 10.1016/j.jpsychires.2015.04.021

Spital, A. (2000, April 27). Evolution of Attitudes at U.S. Transplant Centers Toward Kidney Donation by Friends and Altruistic Strangers. *Transplantation, 69*(8), 1728-1731.

Steury, R. B. (2015, June 18). Non-directed Kidney Donor Rachel Bennett Steury: Paying It Forward. (o. b. Ray Mueller, Interviewer) Retrieved April 21, 2020, from https://www.youtube.com/watch?v=IpCEVnDuORI

Teraoka, R. K. (2009). How Do Living Kidney Donors Develop End-Stage Renal Disease? *American Journal of Transplantation*, 2514-2519. doi:https://onlinelibrary.wiley.com/doi/epdf/10.1111/j.1600-6143.2009.02795.x

The Cleveland Clinic. (2019, April 8). *Dialysis*. Retrieved from The Cleveland Clinic: https://my.clevelandclinic.org/health/treatments/14618-dialysis

The National Institute of Diabetes and Digestive and Kidney Diseases. (n.d.). *Kidney Disease*. Retrieved January 16, 2019, from The National Institute of Diabetes and Digestive and Kidney Diseases: https://www.niddk.nih.gov/health-information/kidney-disease

U.S. Department of Health & Human Services. (n.d.). *Living Non-Directed Organ Donation.* Retrieved January 26, 2026, from Organ Procurement and Transplantation Network: https://optn.transplant.hrsa.gov/resources/ethics/living-non-directed-organ-donation/

U.S. Department of Health and Human Services. (2008). *Partnering with your Transplant Team: A Patient's Guide to Transplantation.* Rockville, MD: U.S. Government Printing Office.

United Network for Organ Sharing. (2005, February 25). *History of living donation.* Retrieved January 23, 2019, from UNOS Transplant Living: https://transplantliving.org/living-donation/history/

United Network for Organ Sharing. (2009). *Living Donation: Information You Need to Know.* Richmond, VA: United Network for Organ Sharing.

Youhana, J. (2012, October 4). Indiana Woman Donates Kidney to Stranger. *The Herald*, p. 6.

Youhana, J. (2012, September 30). Kidney's Gone Heart is Intact. *The Journal Gazette*, p. D1.

# About the Author

Rachel Bennett Steury is originally from the International City of Lorain, Ohio. She currently splits her time between Hawaii, California, and Indiana, where she and her husband foster a thriving conservation habitat. She is "Aunt Rae" to more than forty young people in a big working-class family in the industrial heartland. Rachel specializes in communications for non-profit clients and supports disaster response and relief efforts at the local, state, and national levels.

An alum of the University of Massachusetts-Amherst Labor Center, Indiana University Labor Studies Division, and the Indiana Institute of Technology College of Business, Rachel is a former trade unionist with the United Steelworkers and a member of SOAR, the Steelworkers Organization of Active Retirees. She belongs to the Unitarian Universalist Church of Studio City and is a member of the Authors' Guild, the International Women's Writing Guild, the Association of Writers & Writing Programs, and the Italian American Writers Association.

Rachel's writing has been featured in national outlets such as UU World, Coping with Cancer Magazine, Wildfire Magazine, Surviving Breast Cancer, and Industry Week, and in regional outlets including Honolulu Civil Beat, Indianapolis Business Journal, Building Indiana, Sacramento Bee, Fort Wayne Journal Gazette, The Star, and Valley Scene Magazine. She is the author of the circular "The Real Rachel BS" on Substack, where she writes about family, organ donation, minimalism, breast cancer, Hawai'i Nei, and her Sicilian heritage, among many other topics.

Learn more about the author and her work at bennettsteury.com

# Endnotes

1   (CBS Evening News with Katie Couric, 2010)

2   (Anderson, 2010)

3   (National Kidney Foundation, 2019)

4   (The National Institute of Diabetes and Digestive and Kidney Diseases, n.d.)

5   (Organ Procurement and Transplantation Network, n.d.)

6   (Donate Life America) (Donate Life America)

7   (Organ Procurement and Transplantation Network, n.d.)

8   (United Network for Organ Sharing, 2005)

9   (Organ Procurement and Transplantation Network)

10  (U.S. Department of Health & Human Services)

11  (Organ Procurement and Transplantation Network)

12  (National Kidney Registry, 2019)

13  (Kesner, 2009)

14  (Saulnier)

15  (Khidekel, 2010)

16  (Nutt, 2010)

17  (Graham, 2010)

18  (National Kidney Registry, 2009)

19  (Singer & Lamm, 2009)

20  (National Kidney Registry, 2009)

21  (The Cleveland Clinic, 2019)

22  (Singer P. , 2006)

23  (Milliman Inc., 2008)

24  (Milliman Inc., 2011)

25  (Milliman Inc., 2014)

26  (Milliman Inc., 2017)

27  (Milliman Inc., 2020)

28  (Milliman Inc., 2025)

29  (Ilana Silver Levine & Marian Charlton, 2010)

30  (Fehrman-Ekholm & Groth, 1997)

31  (Goldfarb DA, 2001)

32  (Teraoka, 2009)

33  (National Safety Council, 2019)

34  (Spital, 2000)

35  (Henderson, et al., 2003)

36  (ABC7 Chicago, 2010)

37  (Loyola University Health System, 2010)

38  (Lotus, 2011)

39  (U.S. Department of Health and Human Services, 2008)

40  (United Network for Organ Sharing, 2009)

41  (Annette M. Jackson PhD & Kraus MD)

42  (Annette M. Jackson PhD & Kraus MD)

43  (Cuda-Kroen, 2012)

44  (Andrews, 2002)

45  (Lehman, 2012)

46  (Board, 2013)

47  (Youhana, Kidney's Gone Heart is Intact, 2012)

48  (Youhana, Indiana Woman Donates Kidney to Stranger, 2012)

49  (Sit, 2015)

50  (Bassett K. , 2013)

51  (Donate Life America)

52  (Steury, 2015)

53  (CBS News, 2019)

54  (Gunnerson, 2018)

55  (M. Stadtler, 2005)

56  (Sandler, 1996)

57  (Donate Life Rose Parade Float, 2011)

58  (Donate Life Rose Parade Float, 2018)

59  (Donate Life Rose Parafe Float, 2018)

60  (Bassett K. , 2018)

61  (OneLegacy Foundation, 2019)

62  (OneLegacy, 2019)